JUICE YOUR WAY BACK 10 YEARS

*Let knowledge be your compass
and juice be your fountain of youth*

JUICE
YOUR WAY BACK
10 YEARS
Reverse Aging, Lose Weight, Restore Health,
Regain Energy, and Boost Your Metabolism

**INCLUDES THE MOST EFFECTIVE ANTI-AGING
FRUITS, VEGETABLES, AND HERBAL BLENDS**

JAMES UBERTI

Juice Your Way Back, LLC.

www.juiceyourwayback.com

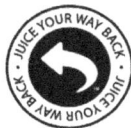

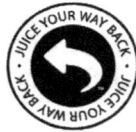

Juice Your Way Back Media
info@juiceyourwayback.com

ISBN

Print version: 978-09970673-9-2

Ebook version: 978-09970673-8-5

First Edition
Printed in the United States of America on acid-free paper.
Cover and Book Design: Bacall Creative

CONTENTS

DISCLAIMER

Please note that much of this publication is based on personal experience and studies. You should use this information as you see fit and at your own risk. Nothing in this book is intended to replace common sense, legal, medical, or other professional advice and is meant solely to inform the reader.

The information provided in this book in no way substitutes for a physician's advice. Please consult with a doctor before conducting any health or juice regimen to avoid any potential problems. For instance, large amounts of foods high in vitamin K, such as kale and spinach, may change how the blood thinner Warfarin works.

No part of this publication may be reproduced or transmitted in any form whatsoever, electronically, or mechanically, including photocopying, recording or by any informational storage or retrieval system without express written, dated, and signed permission from the author.

Juicing is very effective at reversing the signs of premature aging and restoring the body to a healthier state; but don't try drinking it by the gallon thinking it will work faster. When consumed in excess, fruit and vegetable juices can overload the pancreas, kidney, liver and digestive tract. Start slowly. Let your body adjust itself to the way juices work. Then sit back, relax and enjoy the benefits of new energy, vitality, younger looking skin and renewed health and beauty from the inside out.

Because you've been consuming a diet low in fiber, largely consisting of processed foods and toxins you may experience some side effects during this process. Side effects may include but are not limited to headache, upset stomach and some minor body aches. This is normal and will subside as you begin to rid your body of toxins and your body starts to become healthier and more alkaline vs. acidic.

ACKNOWLEDGMENTS

I would like to acknowledge and thank my friends and family for supporting me and encouraging me to follow my dreams, expose the truth, and never give up despite the many obstacles and life lessons learned along the way. I would especially like to thank my mother, a single parent with three children, who taught me the nutritional benefits of a healthy diet and lifestyle. To this day her motherly instincts go into overdrive if, God forbid, I tell her something is wrong with me. She will do extensive research, find a holistic answer, tell me what to eat, what supplement to take, and what juices to blend, even though my response today would be, "Ma, I know. It's my job."

I would like to also thank my friends for supporting me and being role models of happy people, who laugh often and always believe in themselves and set wonderful examples. The true meaning of success is: "To know even one life has breathed easier because you have lived, this is to have succeeded"—Ralph Waldo Emerson. Thank you to those who have allowed me to breath easier. I am forever grateful and blessed.

INTRODUCTION

It's one thing to claim that juicing can help shed pounds as well as nourish and hydrate the body, but what about reverse the signs of aging? Is that possible? Studies are showing that it's very possible, because of the dramatic increase in chemical substitutions in food, environmental toxins, and today's prevailing diet of processed foods. Most humans, if not all, are nutritionally deficient, and lack the essential nutrients necessary to prevent accelerated aging and disease. Chemists and doctors alike agree on one thing—that nutrition, not age, determines the quality of your health and appearance. Nutrition determines everything from the condition of your skin, hair, and nails to the quality of your muscles, connective tissues, bones, and even how effectively your brain functions.

As we age, the collagen that keeps our skin taunt and firm begins to break down, which causes the appearance of wrinkles and sagging skin. These signs of aging normally don't start to occur until after age thirty-five. However, premature aging and wrinkles can still occur. Using expensive lotions, Botox, and plastic surgery to temporarily remove wrinkles is like using a Band-Aid to cover a wound that never heals, because you are only treating the symptoms of aging, not the root cause. Premature aging is due to stress, toxins, sun exposure, weight gain, disease, and damaging free radicals. To treat, slow down and minimize the signs of aging, you need to identify and remove age robbing toxins, balance out your gut bacteria and flood the body with regenerative plant-based foods that revitalize and rejuvenate the body from the inside out.

So throw out your skin creams, anti-aging lotions, and moisturizers that promise to reverse signs of aging. They are a waste of money, and if they do work it's only temporary, and often laden with toxic chemicals that are absorbed into the skin, which can actually cause accelerated aging and disease. The body needs nutrition, not a quick fix, skin treatments, or costly and potentially dangerous surgery. Only proper nutrition and your own body's internal chemistry can produce lasting resiliency in every cell, connective tissue, and organ in the body. Proper education and nutrition are the only things necessary to create healthy cells which can restore, revitalize, and radiate the lasting effects of a youthful appearance and energy, not expensive lotions that claim to give you lasting youth—along with the common dangers of toxic skin creams and lotions.

Think of it this way. Polluting our body with toxic chemicals and denying our bodies of the essential nutrients needed to replace cells, connective tissues, skin, hair and nails rapidly accelerates the aging process. If our bodies lack the essential vitamins, minerals, and enzymes, our cells and organs—which are being replaced every second of every day—become frail, weak, and susceptible to premature aging and disease. The two reasons we get sick, and look and feel older than we are, is simple. Virtually every human being is full of toxins from processed foods and chemicals, and nutritionally deficient in essential vitamins, minerals, and enzymes. The main problem is food corporations and product manufacturers aren't required to disclose the facts about the dangers of the toxic ingredients they use or their effects on the body. It's not until there are class action lawsuits filed and/or media attention that we find out that dangerous chemicals are used. We lack the knowledge to even find out what's making us sick and tired and aging us prematurely. In my book you will learn the toxic truth about what corporations don't want you to know, from the foods you eat, to the products you use, to the water you drink. Such things are aging us at an alarming rate, and causing widespread disease and death.

All processed foods and meats are full of toxic chemicals that are then stored in our bodies, slowing down our ability to lose weight, eliminate waste, and revitalize cells. Those toxins are what age us prematurely.

You will learn the truth about what happens behind the scenes, before food is delivered and packaged with enticing often-misleading advertisements on the packaging. For example, if a food item says non-fat, food manufacturers often add chemicals and/or artificial sweeteners as a substitute for trans fats or saturated fats, both to make it taste good and to get you addicted to the chemicals. Did you know that farm-raised salmon are fed processed pellets that contain soybeans, chicken fat, and ground feathers? This diet turns the salmon's flesh grey. Dye is then used to color the salmon pink to make it look like wild-caught salmon, according to an article in *The Atlantic* in March of 2015. Wild salmon get their pink skin color from krill in the ocean, not chemical dye like farm-raised salmon. Did you know that 79% of tuna served in sushi restaurants isn't even tuna but a substitute fish called Escolar, which resembles mackerel and has the texture of tuna? Did you know that trans fats and hydrogenated oils are among the worst offenders in premature aging and disease, and are found in most baked goods, snacks, fried foods, and coffee creamers? These chemicals significantly increase the body's inflammation, raising bad cholesterol (LDL) and lowering good cholesterol (HDL) as the chemicals attack collagen in your body, causing the skin to wrinkle and produce age spots.

In this book I expose the truth about what foods, products, and toxins to avoid, empower you with the knowledge to identify age-robbing culprits, and show you how to flood your body with superfoods and juice blends that revitalize, restore, and reverse the signs of premature aging from the inside out. I will educate you on the chemicals that are hidden and considered dangerous in our food and water, and in products you use every day. I list the most effective fruits, vegetables, and herbal blends to cleanse and nourish your body, and give your cells the necessary nutrients needed to repair your appearance and bring back that youthful glow. I will teach you which antioxidant-rich fruits, vegetables, and herbs to eat to neutralize your acidic body to achieve a healthy, PH-balanced internal chemistry. Everything in life must be in balance to function properly. The oceans for example are very similar to our bodies. If it becomes out of balance from toxic pollution and global warming, coral and fish (represented of our cells in our body) start to become weak, diseased and die. A diet high in healthy PH alkaline-based foods, probiotics, and enzymes can put harmony and balance back in your life and help fight and resist disease, give you more energy, boost your mood, and give you a youthful glow and energy for life.

Let's face it: most people want to look attractive, and of course doing also so boosts our self-image, gives us confidence, and helps us become more successful both personally and professionally. In fact, in a recent study, facial plastic surgery is on the rise due in part to our obsession with "selfies" and social media. There's no denying that social media platforms like Facebook, Instagram and "selfie" iPhone apps are pushing us to put ourselves under the microscope, making us more self-conscious about our appearances than ever before.

Companies in the beauty, dietary, and medical industries take advantage of our self-obsessed society to blast you with marketing messages, hoping that you will be deceived into thinking that if you buy this, take that, and use this, you will magically feel and look younger—virtually overnight. And that message is all around us. We are saturated by ads and commercials that run morning, noon and night. Unfortunately, we live in a "looks matter" world. Even if you personally feel you have moved beyond this, your outside appearance is nonetheless a huge part of your life, impacting everything from landing a job to attracting a partner. The good news is that wellness and radiant skin rarely involve radical, unsustainable changes if you're educated about the facts, and are sincerely committed to making a difference in your health and appearance. It is my belief that your life will be better every single day through small, simple, hand-to-mouth healthy choices. Many elements of life begin to fall into place when we give our bodies the care they deserve. When you treat your body well, your mind, skin, and emotions all benefit.

Removing toxins, balancing your body's PH and gut health and juicing will greatly diminish or reverse the signs of aging, restore your health, and give you the body and youthful appearance you desire. It's scary how easy and attainable this is. Simply follow the steps outlined in my book. You are the driver of this new journey. However, you must believe. You must be committed. You must be committed, stay the course and follow the advice given in my book, by doing so; I guarantee a life of better health and a younger-looking appearance that will be noticed and envied by coworkers, friends, and family.

Individuals who have undertaken our *Juice Your Way Back* chal-lenge for twenty or even forty days have seen nothing short of a transformation, a jump backward in time to a younger, leaner, healthier self. Two things happened as they followed the advice given in my book. First, they dramatically reduced their toxin intake. Second, they flooded their bodies with plant-based nutrients and probiotics, resulting in dramatic weight loss, increased vitality and energy, clearer mind and mood, as well as a more youthful and healthier appearance, undoing years of damage from an unhealthy age-robbing lifestyle.

ABOUT THE AUTHOR

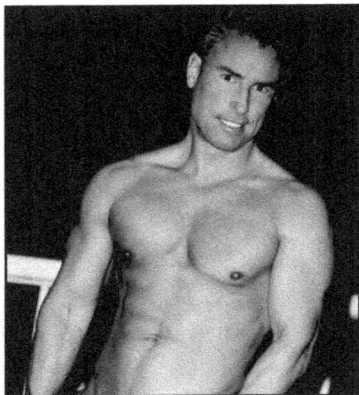

The inspiration for the *Juice Your Way Back* books and rejuvenation juice blends came from fifty-one years young founder James Uberti, certified holistic nutritionist, triathlete, entrepreneur, trainer, motivational speaker, and fitness enthusiast for over thirty years. During that time, I met many individuals who struggled to lose weight and get in shape. Even if they achieved their weight loss goal, they often gained it back again. This extra weight caused them to look sick, tired, and older than their actual age. That was when it hit me. There had to be a better way to get in shape and lose weight, keep it off, and reverse the signs of aging at the same time. Fast-forward several years later. After extensive research, and after personally experimenting with several types of superfoods, herbal blends, and juice recipes, the *Juice Your Way Back* books and blends were born.

In my late teens, I became involved in bodybuilding competitions. After my third competition, I decided that competitive bodybuilding was not the career path for me, although health and fitness have continued to be my passion. My belief now that I recently turned 51 years young is that if you invest in your health, the second half of your life can be the very best years ahead. That being said, throughout my life I have lived a healthy lifestyle, eating right and exercising regularly. Over a decade ago, while training for my first triathlon, I began experiencing heart palpitations, dizziness, and nausea. After several trips to the emergency room, I was diagnosed with an abnormal heart rhythm (hearth arrhythmia), caused by physical and mental stress, high blood pressure, high triglycerides levels, and low levels of electrolytes.

That was my turning point. I began incorporating low sugar, plant-based foods into my diet. In a short time, my condition improved dramatically, and after several months of juicing at least once a day, I started noticing the positive side effects. My skin looked better. I was leaner. I had more energy and increased stamina. I never got sick. Overall, I felt and looked younger than I had in years. After years of following this same regime, I often get compliments on how fit and youthful I look for my age. I welcome the idea of living longer and love the idea of looking and feeling ten to twenty years younger, being healthy, clear-minded and energetic well into my sixties, seventies, eighties, and beyond.

Let knowledge be your compass
and juice be your fountain of youth.

CHAPTER 1

WE AGE FROM
THE INSIDE OUT

Diet and nutrition, not the number of candles on your birthday cake, determine how you feel on the inside and look on the outside. Your body's internal chemistry dictates, in large part, the quality and resiliency of virtually every cell and organ in your body. There may be up to 32,000,000,000,000 cells (yes, 32 trillion!) in the human body. For the most part, your cells, body parts, bones, hair, skin, and organs are all replaced several times throughout your lifetime. This process is called regenerative cell replacement. Toxins from the food we eat to the products we use contribute to how slow or fast we age or become sick and greatly affecting the quality of your skin to the efficiency of organs in the body.

When cells don't get the right food and nutrients from your diet, they become weak, tired, and die prematurely. If you don't change your diet, the new replacement cells will be just as weak as the old ones. Think of it this way. If you were building a house and chose the cheapest, weakest building materials to build your new home, how long do you think it would last? Your body is the same way. The food and water you consume determines the strength and resiliency of every cell in your body. As a result, your eating habits are a major determinant in how quickly you begin to see and feel the effects of aging. Each cell in your body needs vital vitamins, minerals, and enzymes to replace disease-resistant cells. Depriving your body of these essential repair materials will weaken your immune system, and your body will show signs of premature aging at an alarming rate. Toxins contribute to a weak immune system and greatly effect the appearance of the skin.

Today, the typical American diet includes too many inflamma-tory toxic foods that undermine skin, nail, and hair health. Cellular inflammation, or micro-inflammation, breaks down the skin cells and the body's supply of collagen, destroying elasticity and eventu-ally resulting in wrinkles and sallow, sagging skin. Highly processed foods, common in our fast food diets, can hasten aging by creat-ing protein-like substances called peptides and neuropeptides that increase this inflammatory and collagen-damaging process.

Aging is inevitable. But the rate at which your skin ages, as well as its overall health, can be dramatically slowed and even reversed. This type of aging is not chronological, but cellular, called biological aging. In other words, we age from the inside out, one cell at a time.

Mitochondria are fuel factories in our cells that convert the food we eat into energy. When mitochondria malfunction, cells die. How well we age, including our vulnerability to disease, is due in part to how healthy our mitochondria are. Recent studies have linked oxidative stress—the accumulation of free radicals in the cell—and genetic defects in mitochondria with premature aging.

And what causes mitochondria to malfunction and die? Systemic inflammation in the body. A common cause of inflammation is a high-sugar diet. Too much sugar or high-glycemic food ultimately leads to a metabolic process called glycation (or glycosylation) in which sugar molecules in the blood bond to proteins and DNA, which over time become chemically modified. These newly bonded proteins are called AGEs, or advanced glycation end products. AGEs create unnatural cross-links with collagen proteins. This changes their shape, flexibility, elasticity, and function. The result is premature aging. What's more, the presence of AGEs gener-ates additional inflammation. Inflammation and glycation are two related reactions that impact the body's natural state of balance and manifest themselves as aging throughout the body's organ systems, most visibly in the skin.

Scientists claim they have evidence to explain why diet, exercise, and reducing stress can reverse the aging effects of a poor diet and sedentary lifestyle. Based on a small, exploratory study, researchers say these good habits work by preventing chromosomes in our cells from unraveling. Basically, they assert that healthy living can reverse the effects of aging on a genetic level. It relates to the little caps on our chromosomes called telomeres. They work like the plastic tips of shoelaces to protect the ends of chromosomes, which are the strings of genes in the heart of every cell that tell it what to do. Without telomeres, our cells would lose the ability to divide and would quickly die off.

Scientists have been fascinated by telomeres for decades. In 2009, Elizabeth Blackburn shared a Nobel Prize for pioneering work in the field. What she discovered was that, as living things age, their telomeres get shorter and shorter—a well-grounded observation that some scientists think is not only a marker of aging but a fundamental driver of premature aging and senility. Smoking, poor diet, stress, and lack of exercise are driving factors to making telomeres shorter which leads to a greater risk of accelerated aging, chronic diseases and a shorter lifespan.

Those in the study group that included a healthy diet, low in fats, sugars, and processed foods, walked for an hour a day and performed stress management techniques, including yoga and meditation for an hour a day, and spending more time with friends and family, found over time that the length of their telomeres increased by 10%.

Proof positive that stress, poor diet and lack of exercise can in fact accelerate the aging process down to the cellular level.

The good news is that you can reverse this effect. Your body is an amazing organism. All it wants to do is heal, thrive, and survive. Once you understand what robs your body of its health and vitality, and what to do about it, you are well on your way to looking and feeling much younger. In the next couple of chapters you will learn the toxic truth about foods, chemicals, and pesticides that are aging us prematurely and making us susceptible to disease and death.

CHAPTER 2

AGE-ROBBING CULPRITS

Foods, Fats, Drugs and Parasites

If your diet includes vegetable oils, margarine, processed meats, white bread, sugar, processed foods, and "fast foods," you're not doing your body or appearance any favors. These foods can cause inflammation in your body, which accelerates wrinkle formation. Processed food and "fast food" offer only empty calories that are nutritionally void, toxic, chemically designed to be addictive, and actually accelerate the aging process and promote disease.

Our bodies naturally produce human growth hormone (HGH) in the pituitary gland. Among its many functions, HGH works with collagen to maintain skin and muscle composition. As we age, our body's natural production of collagen slows, which can lead to looser and thinner skin. While you may not be able to stop time completely in its tracks, you *can* reverse these effects by eliminating the foods, toxins, and chemicals that accelerate the aging process, and flood your cells with antioxidant-rich superfoods instead. These provide every cell with the essential building blocks to restore and replace old cells with stronger and more resilient ones.

If you deprive your body of essential nutrients, vitamins, enzymes and minerals by eating a nutrient-void diet, it's like calling in demolition crews but never calling the construction crews. Of course, the occasional processed food or hamburger with a side of fries isn't going to turn you into Rip Van Winkle, but when dietary lapses become daily habits, they can erase years from your skin, life, and put you at risk of disease.

In recent decades, processed food, "fast food," and convenience food consumption in the United States have increased dramatically. More than 35% of people are now consuming diets of predominantly junk food. This trend has occurred concurrently with rising epidemics of chronic diseases, such as obesity.

By the year 2050, the rate of obesity in the U.S. is expected to reach alarming rates, according to researchers at Harvard University. Children who eat processed food regularly consume more fat, carbohydrates, and processed sugar—and virtually no fiber—than those who do not eat "fast food" regularly. Obesity increases your risk for cardiovascular disease and diabetes, and accelerates the aging process dramatically. As the largest organ in your body, the skin is the last to show signs of a diseased body.

When eating processed foods and sugars, your insulin levels are elevated due to the presence of high fructose corn syrups or processed and/or artificial sweeteners and sugars. Examples of this are soft drinks, white flour, and other foods devoid of fiber and nutrients necessary to properly metabolize carbohydrates. Eating junk food throughout the day causes chronically high insulin levels, which eventually prompt your cells to begin to ignore this important hormone. This results in a condition known as insulin resistance.

Processed foods and overgrowth of bad intestinal bacteria lead to depression in both children and adults, and make you more susceptible to mood and behavioral swings. This effect is especially prevalent in teens, since foods high in fat cause hormone imbalances and irregularities. Consuming trans fats, saturated fats, and processed foods is associated with up to a 58% increase in risk of depression. It's no surprise that antidepressant, ADHD, and bipolar medications are the number one prescribed drugs in this country. The second and third most commonly prescribed drugs are for acid reflux and blood thinners. Conditions all caused by toxic diets high in sugar, salt, and fats, and devoid of nutrients and fiber.

High sodium levels are often characteristic of many processed foods, and one of the contributing factors to the overconsumption of salt. Salt is ever-present in a Western diet, and contributes to high blood pressure and heart, liver, and kidney diseases, according to Harvard Health Publications. The average American eats five to **ten times** more salt than the 2,300 milligrams per day recommended by the U.S. Dietary Guidelines. Considering the high rates of high blood pressure among Americans, that level should be even lower—about 1,500 milligrams per day—for 70% of adults.

One of the biggest challenges today is not having enough time to get everything done, let alone plan for and choose a healthy lifestyle. We are so busy that we often sacrifice our health for convenient "fast food" choices. In addition, we often wait until the last minute to feed ourselves, when hunger is at its greatest peak and our bodies say "feed me now."

When this happens, we reach for the quickest options to satisfy or alleviate hunger pains, which causes us to overeat every time. What makes it worse, the hormone or trigger that says "hey, you're full" is often suppressed or delayed, which often causes us to overeat. These triggers are delayed because of the consumption of unhealthy fats and oils that, when absorbed, interfere with communication between your stomach and brain.

Below is a list of ingredients that accelerate premature aging

Trans Fat (A vegetable oil concoction infused with hydrogen atoms.)

How It Ages You: Trans fat significantly accelerates the aging process in numerous ways, but let's start with the most harmful result—inflammation. Trans fat is to chronic inflammation what gasoline is to fire. Inflammation ages you from the inside out by damaging your cells, causing free radical production and nibbling away at your telomeres. The length of telomeres is not only a sign of how old you are, but also a measurement of how well your body is aging. The shorter the telomeres the less effectively it regenerates your organs.

Trans fat also adds years to your age by dulling the communication between cells. Yes, Cells in fact communicate with each other through their own language of chemical signals. Different compounds, such as hormones and neurotransmitters, act like words and phrases, telling a cell about the environment around it or communicating messages. Cells need pliable walls to communicate with one another.

The body makes cell walls out of fat—good fat equals healthy walls; bad fat equals unstable walls. Because trans fat is man-made, the molecule has an unnatural shape. "Like forcing a square peg into a round hole, trans fat's odd dimension gums up the system," says Kevin Spelman, PhD, a research scientist in the Department of Biochemistry at the University of North Carolina at Greensboro. "On a very core level, the odd shape begins to change cell-to-cell signaling and membrane fluidity which has a profound effect on both your overall health and aging."

Foods that Contain Trans Fats: Canned biscuits and cinnamon rolls often contain trans fats, as do frozen pizza crusts. Non-dairy coffee creamers, stick margarines, French fries, anything fried or battered, pie and pie crust, shortening, cakes mixes and frostings, pancakes and waffles, cookies, breakfast sandwiches, ground beef, canned chili, frozen or creamy beverages, Asian crunchy noodles, and packaged pudding.

The Dangers of Trans Fats: Trans fat is known to increase blood levels of low density lipoprotein (LDL), or "bad" cholesterol, while lowering levels of high density lipoprotein (HDL), known as "good" cholesterol. It can also cause the arteries to clog, type 2 diabetes, and increase the risk of other serious health problems, such as heart disease. Many food companies use trans fat instead of oil because it reduces cost, extends storage life of products, and can improve flavor and texture.

But those companies are not required to list trans fat on nutrition labels, so consumers have no way of knowing how much trans fat is in the food they eat. Furthermore, there is no upper safety limit recommended for the daily intake of trans fat. The Food and Drug Administration (FDA) has said only that your "intake of trans fats should be as low as possible."

One tip to determine the amount of trans fat in a food is to read the ingredient label and look for shortening, hydrogenated or partially hydrogenated oil. The higher up on the list these ingredients appear, the more trans fat there is in the product.

You can also add up the amount of fat in a product (saturated, monounsaturated and polyunsaturated), provided the amounts are listed, and compare the total with the total fat on the label. If they don't match up, the difference is likely trans fat, especially if partially hydrogenated oil is one of the first ingredients listed.

A few companies, like Frito Lay, Lipton, and Nestle, have already taken steps to eliminate trans fat in some products. Nestle is removing it from several of their products. Their competitor, Cadbury, is also considering removing trans fats from some of its products, as is Kraft.

A lawsuit was recently filed against Nabisco, the Kraft Foods unit that makes Oreo cookies, seeking a ban on the sale of Oreo cookies because they contain trans fat, making them dangerous to eat. The case was later withdrawn because the lawyer who filed the suit said the publicity surrounding the case accomplished what he set out to do: create awareness about the dangers of trans fat.

Hydrogenated Oil (A chemical process in which hydrogen is added to liquid oils and a catalyst metal such as nickel.)

How It Ages You: Hydrogenated oil and vegetable oils are highly perishable, and when heated or exposed to light or moisture, they undergo a toxic change called oxidation. Oxidation can stimulate several age-related diseases. Oxidation is aging. Oxidized oils attack collagen, causing skin to wrinkle and produce age spots. These brown skin spots often form on the face, the backs of the hands, and in organs such as the heart by attacking the artery walls and causing heart disease. They also attack the liver, spleen, kidneys, gallbladder, and intestines, causing these organs to operate less efficiently. The major issue is that the body doesn't recognize this man-maid synthetic process and has a difficult time digesting the molecules, causing them to remain in your body longer. This can cause chronic age-related in inflammation, digestive problems, and weight gain.

Foods that contain Hydrogenated Oils: Margarine, vegetable shortening, non-dairy whipped dessert topping, cake frosting, white bread, non-dairy coffee creamers, tortillas, fast food, hot dogs, hot dog buns, donuts, peanut butter, and ice cream.

Dangers of Hydrogenated Oil: Hydrogenated oils contribute to high cholesterol by scarring the internal walls of the arteries. This is due to the metal (usually nickel) often used in the hydrogenation process. This causes the body to produce cholesterol to repair the walls of the arteries, which is one reason plaque can build up on the arterial walls. Continuous scarring slowly shrinks the area that blood flows through, forcing the heart work much harder and faster, eventually wearing it out. This thicker blood also has a harder time pumping through the arteries and brain. Ever get dizzy, feel faint, or have brain fog? That's why.

It can also cause Alzheimer's, Parkinson's, ADHD, and muddled thinking, just to name a few. Remember too that one of the metals sometimes used in the hydrogenation process is aluminum, which has been linked to the onset of Alzheimer's disease in a number of studies.

One story I read was about a surgeon, who performed surgery on an overweight patient and found a thick, fatty substance in patient's arteries. This was later identified as the fatty, hydrogenated, oil-laden, fast food breakfast the patient had eaten the day before surgery.

Not a pleasant thought at all. Hydrogenated oils are great as preservatives precisely because all the enzymatic activity in the oil has been neutralized during the hydrogenating process. This hydrogenated oil is only one molecule away from plastic, and plastic does not break down in the human body. It lasts for millennia, which is one reason that even our oceans are starting to turn into plastic wastelands. If hydrogenated oils were not used, most foods would spoil very quickly. That's because natural oils have enzymatic activity, which is what causes them and all foods to go bad at room temperature. Any food that does not rot at room temperature is considered a "dead" food and should not be consumed.

In fact, the faster a food goes bad, the healthier it usually is. That's because the enzymatic activity, which causes it to spoil at room temperature, also means that the enzymatic activity within your own body will be greater. Food is basically meant to digest itself, so eating foods high in natural enzymes such as fresh vegetables, fruits, and other raw foods means less stress on your digestive system.

The more enzyme dead processed foods and ingredients you consume, the more your body has to create and use up its own food enzymes during digestion, causing the entire body stress, but especially the pancreas, which has to create the necessary food enzymes for digestion. This is even more difficult, and the body never truly digests these kinds of foods, because they are not a substance that the body is designed to absorb or break down. Such foreign substances often cause false immune responses, which can strain the immune system and decrease overall health.

As the body sends more enzymes (digestive acids) into the stomach to try and digest this plastic-like oil, the internal stomach temperature rises. This is how these unhealthy oils can lead to cancer. It can take thousands of degrees to break down plastic. The body is often only partially successful at breaking down and digesting hydrogenated oils.

To help avoid hydrogenated oils, most of your foods should be raw, juiced, or blended and as close to their natural state as possible. This means more fruits and vegetables, including organic local meats as fresh as possible. The more real foods from nature that you eat, the less packaged and processed foods you'll consume.

Because you can't rely on the government to tell you what is safe to put into your body, you must absolutely become a label reader and check every packaged or processed food you buy. You especially want to make sure that hydrogenated oils and other negative ingredients such as high fructose corn syrup are not listed as ingredients, even on packages that have the word "organic" on the box.

They're not truly healthy if they have additional ingredients that you don't recognize. To be truly healthy, a food must be full of enzymes and phytonutrients, with all their natural vitamins and minerals present. Enzymes are biological molecules that speed up the rate of virtually all of the chemical reactions that take place within a cell. Enzymes are found in melons, mangos, kiwi, grapes, avocado, raw honey, wheat grass juice and coconut water. Enzymes are actually more important than any vitamin, mineral, or other nutrient since all processes that occur in the body must have sufficient supplies of enzymes to happen. Foods that have had their enzymes destroyed though processing or heat are automatically classified as "dead foods."

And eating out can pose just as great a health risk as packaged and processed foods. That's because many restaurants use hydrogenated oils in nearly everything they prepare. The best solution is to purchase organic raw foods and juice at home as often as you can, and get as far away from a processed food diet as possible. Seek out organic superfoods for those times you're on-the-go and need to refuel, as opposed to fast food or processed food. This way, you know exactly what you're putting into your body and not leaving it up to modern manufacturers of today's so called "Frankenfoods," which are often made with addictive chemical additives and toxic flavor enhancers. Remember, food manufacturers aren't tightly regulated by the FDA, and food mislabeling and fraud is rampant nationwide.

Sugar/Sucrose (The refined, highly-processed and crystallized version of plant sugars.)

These consist of any form of processed sugar, high fructose corn syrup, cane juice, malt syrup, and any word ending in "ose," such as glucose. Every one of these types of sugars produces carbohydrates. These age-robbing demons are often disguised as carbs.

Foods that contain starchy carbohydrates: most breads, crackers, chips, cookies, cakes, muffins, pancakes, pies, candy, breaded or battered foods, most cereals, pastas, bagels, pizza, puddings, jellies, jams and preserves, granola bars, power bars, energy bars, tortillas (unless 100% stone-ground whole grain), fried foods, ketchup, sweetened yogurts, and any type of sweetened dairy products, sodas, or carbonated or energy drinks.

How It Ages You: The human body evolved with a finite ability to break down refined sugar and very limited access to it in concentrated forms. This means that processing the comparatively giant loads we consume on a daily basis puts a huge strain on our systems. Excess sugar drifts into the blood, and causes trouble by latching onto protein molecules in an age-accelerating process called glycosylation which, in turn, causes cellular aging in several ways.

First, it slows down the body's repair mechanism. Although glycosylation's effects are mostly internal, aging skin is a prime external sign. When too much sugar in the blood causes glycosylation, the skin loses its natural repair mechanisms, as explained by Shawn Talbott, PhD, a nutritional biochemist and author of *The Metabolic Method* (Currant Book, 2008). "Sugar molecules gum up the collagen in your skin," he writes, "which makes it less elastic, makes it wrinkle faster, and means it won't heal as quickly if it's damaged."

Glycosylation is the process by which sugars are chemically attached to proteins to form glycoproteins, and ages the body by spawning oxidative stress. Sugar molecules cut and irritate everything they touch like shards of glass, says Dr. Mehmet Oz. The damage, called oxidation, eventually leads to a buildup of toxins called AGEs (short for advanced glycation end products). The accumulation of some AGEs is natural—other significant sources of AGEs are meats cooked at high temperatures, such as bacon, hot dogs, or beef. And AGEs in the blood increase fivefold during a person's lifetime—but eating poorly is like hitting the fast-forward button on aging and disease.

Dangers of Sugar

In order to understand the dangers of sugar, you need to understand what it's made of. Before table sugar enters the bloodstream from the digestive tract, it is broken down into two simple sugars—glucose and fructose. **Glucose** is found in every living cell on the planet. If we don't get it from our diet, our bodies produce it. **Fructose** is different. Our bodies do not produce it in any significant amount, and there is no physiological need for it.

Our livers cannot metabolize fructose in any significant amounts. Although fruits contain fructose it is advised to eat or juice fruits in smaller amounts than vegetables. However it's almost impossible to get too much fructose by eating fruit. Once consumed fructose is turned into glycogen and stored in the liver until we need it. However, if the liver is full of glycogen (much more common), eating a lot of processed fructose overloads the liver, forcing it to turn the fructose into fat.

When large amounts of sugar are consumed repeatedly, this process can lead to a fatty liver and other serious problems. When fructose gets turned into fat in the liver, it is shipped out as VLDL cholesterol particles. However, not all of the fat gets out; some of it can lodge in the liver. This can lead to non-alcoholic fatty liver disease (NAFLD), a increasing problem associated with metabolic diseases. Recent studies show that individuals with fatty livers consume up to 2 to 3 times more fructose as the average person.

Insulin is a very important hormone in the body. It allows glucose (blood sugar) to enter cells from the bloodstream and tells the cells to start burning glucose instead of fat. One feature of the metabolic dysfunction caused by the typical Western diet is that insulin stops working as it should. The cells become resistant to it. This insulin resistance is believed to be a leading driver of many diseases… including metabolic syndrome, obesity, cardiovascular disease and **especially** type II diabetes.

Many studies show that sugar consumption is associated with insulin resistance, especially when it is consumed in large amounts. Having too much glucose in the blood is **highly toxic** and one of the reasons for complications of diabetes, which can also lead to blindness and many other diseases caused by too much sugar in your diet.

Starchy Carbohydrates (Refined, processed carbs stripped all of life-giving vitamins and minerals.)

How It Ages You: Refined carbs are sugars in disguise. Every starch turns into sugar the minute it hits your bloodstream. Beyond glycosylation, refined carbs set the stage for insulin resistance.

After a meal laden with refined carbohydrates, the body's blood-sugar levels soar, and the pancreas sprays insulin into the bloodstream to help cells convert the food's energy (glucose) into fuel. The body, however, often miscalculates and releases too much insulin, because (again) evolution hasn't kept pace with the modern diet. If you consume four to five slices of white bread, that's the food-density equivalent to eating a deer. Your body reacts with a massive surge of chemicals to digest all the stuff it thinks you just ate.

As a result of too much insulin, blood-sugar levels drop, and thirty minutes later you're hungry again. The body wasn't designed for this yo-yo effect. All it can do is break apart in bits and pieces. The technical term for this effect is insulin resistance, a precursor to such age-related diseases such as type 1 and type 2 diabetes, metabolic syndrome, and heart disease.

Type 2 diabetes results from the body having high insulin levels for too long. Insulin is meant to be a fast-acting hormone—you release it when glucose levels are high to make them drop. Then the signal stops. If you constantly eat too much or have a very sugary diet, you can end up with high insulin levels all the time. This leads to the body becoming desensitized to insulin. Type 2 diabetes is that much more dangerous because the body will rarely respond to insulin treatment, meaning that drastic diet changes and exercise are the only ways to fight back.

Insulin regulation is one of the most important factors in health in the human body, and yet most people don't really understand why our bodies make it or how what we eat affects the levels of insulin we produce. More so than any hormone, our diet is key in regulating insulin levels, and thus a number of biological processes.

Foods that spike insulin production: most breads, crackers, chips, cookies, cakes, muffins, pancakes, pies, candy, breaded or battered foods, most cereals, pastas, bagels, pizza, puddings, jellies, jams and preserves, granola bars, power bars, energy bars, tortillas (unless 100% stone-ground whole grain), fried foods, ketchup, sweetened yogurts, and any type of sweetened dairy products, sodas, or any carbonated or energy drinks.

Dangers of Starchy Carbohydrate Foods: As mentioned earlier, simple and complex carbs produce the same results sugar does when the body breaks it down into sugar. Eating carbs *and* sugars essentially doubles the amount of inflammation and stress put on your body. Both stimulate the pleasure sensors of the brain— in fact, just thinking about sugar or carbs triggers the pleasure sensors in the brain. This is due to the addictive properties of both substances, which makes you want to eat more than you need. Excess starch and sugar are easily converted to fat, especially when accompanied by high insulin levels brought about by increased blood sugar levels.

First you will need to follow the steps outlined below on how to detox the body and flood it instead with life-giving, age-reversing superfoods, herbs, and blends. Carbohydrates are necessary for fuel, so to get the small amount of carbs needed, substitute starchy foods with fruits, nuts, seeds, and their butters.

High Fructose Corn Syrup (As the name implies, it is made from corn, then milled to produce starch—corn starch, or corn syrup whose glucose has been partially changed into fructose.)

How It Ages You: There's often talk about the negative effects of eating sugary food, but just as dangerous as sugar is high fructose corn syrup (HFCS), which is often hidden in processed food and sodas. Unlike sugar, HFCS does not break down properly in the body. HFCS causes weight gain and stresses the liver by forcing it to work harder.

Your skin also reacts to HFCS, which causes a host of problems, mainly acne. Long-term effects of HFCS consumption include premature aging and scarring. As mentioned earlier, sugar attaches to proteins in the bloodstream, forming new molecules called advanced glycation end products (AGEs) that damage both collagen and elastin, which contributes to sagging and premature wrinkling. AGEs also deactivate natural antioxidant enzymes, leaving the skin more susceptible to sun damage.

Foods that contain high fructose corn syrup: juice cocktails, soda, breakfast cereal, yogurt, salad dressing, breads and baked goods, candy and candy bars, health bars, breads, beverages, breakfast pastries, condiments, cough syrups, crackers, dairy, drink mixers, canned fruits and vegetables, ice cream, jams, jellies, syrups, meats, pastries, steak sauce, and soups.

Dangers of High Fructose Corn Syrup: Consumption of high-fructose corn syrup can lead to a significant increase in the likelihood of developing pre- and post-type 1 and type 2 diabetes. You can either avoid diabetes or reverse the condition with knowledge and hand-to-mouth choices every day. The good news is that this can be avoided and/or reversed if educated on the dangers of age-robbing toxins and processed foods and flooding your cells with food that is used to make stronger more reliant ones.

If you drink sodas, **stop!** If you drink energy drinks, **stop!** If you eat junk food, **stop!** Otherwise, you may be faced with losing a foot or going blind or living with diabetes. High-fructose corn syrup doesn't just make your body fat, it also makes your heart fat and diseased, and accelerates aging and damages cells.

There is a strong link between the consumption of high fructose corn syrup and elevated triglyceride and LDL (bad cholesterol) levels. Combined, these can cause arterial plaque build-up and lead to heart problems including hypertension, heart disease, accelerated cell damage, even strokes. Your liver, gallbladder, and kidneys process toxins and HFCS are especially destructive to your liver. When combined with a sedentary life-style, permanent liver scarring can occur. When combined with a sedentary lifestyle, permanent liver scarring can occur. This greatly diminishes the organ's ability to process toxins and, over time, can lead to a range of major negative health effects, not just grey, saggy skin, and acne. If that's not enough to convince you to change your intake levels, did you know high fructose corn syrup is often loaded with alarmingly high levels of mercury? One study found mercury in over 50% of samples tested, according to article in *Global Health* on the dangers of HFCS. Mercury exposure can result in irreversible brain and nervous system damage—especially in children.

Ghrelin (A hormone made by the digestive system that increases appetite and tells your body it's hungry.)

How It Ages You: Waiting too long between meals is one of the surest ways to age the body before its time. That's because hunger pains may lead to choosing fast food, or to eating too much food. A hungry stomach sends "feed me now" signals to the brain by releasing the hormone ghrelin. The problem is that it takes around thirty minutes for ghrelin levels to return to normal once you've started eating, which of course leads to overeating. In addition, researchers have discovered that high levels of saturated fats and trans fats either mask or delay that "fullness" signal, causing us to overeat.

No one eats perfectly all the time. Occasional digressions aren't worth stressing. But arming yourself with facts and making small changes can lead to a healthier mind, body, and spirit.

Cortisol (A stress hormone secreted by the adrenal glands.)

How It Ages You: Stress hormones—automatically released by the body under all kinds of stressful circumstances—are antithetical to digestion in several ways. First, the release of adrenaline and cortisol—"fight-or-flight" chemicals—diverts blood toward your limbs and away from your stomach and intestines, which hinders your intestines' ability to break down food and absorb nutrients. As a result, digestion grinds to a halt, and food ferments, sending unusual metabolites into the bloodstream, explains Kevin Spelman, PhD, a research scientist in the Department of Biochemistry at the University of North Carolina in Greensboro.

Second, stress throws off the gut's acidity and its ability to absorb certain nutrients, such as vitamin B12. As if that weren't enough, cortisol also suppresses the body's natural repair mechanisms. "By eating when you're stressed, it's as if you are damaging your body and locking out the repair crews," says Henry Lodge, MD, co-author of the New York Times best-seller *Younger Next Year: Live Strong, Fit and Sexy—Until You're 80 and Beyond* (Workman Publishing, 2004). Eating while stressed or distracted also makes you vulnerable to eating more than you intended, and prone to eating foods you wouldn't have under better circumstances.

Trying to look your best, be healthy, fit, and disease-free is becoming more and more difficult in a world that is becoming more and more toxic. Despite the attention of the health profession, the media, the public, and despite educational campaigns about the benefits of a healthier diet and increased physical activity, we are headed toward disaster. According to the American Diabetes Association, the obesity rate in the United States has more than doubled over the past four decades. We, as a nation, practice the habits of "super-sizing," speed, and convenience.

In addition, processed food manufacturers and "fast food" chains are using technology to process foods that are addictive, chemical-laden, full of preservatives and God knows what else. Food manufacturers spend hundreds of millions of dollars on focus groups and marketing tricks to get you to impulsively purchase their products. For example, when food manufacturers learned that consumers wanted to eat a low-fat or no-fat diet, they quickly changed their addictive fat formulas and substituted fat with sugar. The problem was by taking out the fat the product tasted bland, by adding sugar it taste great and sugar is highly addictive, which, if not burned off, converts to fat much faster then had they left the fat in the product in the first place.

Processed food manufacturers and fast food chains use sugar, salt, fat, and chemical additives to get you addicted, and cheaper, toxic ingredients to increase their profits. Depending on where you get your fast food fix, the calorie count in a regular to "super-sized" meal is often off-the-charts high, and the sugar, salt, and fat levels more than likely exceed what your body can process and eliminate. These three ingredients are known as trigger substances, meaning when all three are combined into a food, they keep you coming back for more until your body becomes addicted. This addiction spikes when other flavor enhancers are added into the mix.

"Most people don't realize how very sedentary their life has become," says Steven N. Blair, PED (physical education doctor), director of research at The Cooper Institute in Dallas. According to Dr. Blair, a major (and often unrecognized) reason for Americans' widening waistlines is this "gradual ratcheting down of daily life activity." The average adult expends about 300-700 fewer calories per day than their parents did, he says.

Even if you eat well and are diligent about making healthy food choices, you still may not be getting an adequate amount of certain nutrients that help aid in healthier looking skin, hair, and nails, thanks to several factors that interfere with absorption of essential nutrients that promote health, vitality, and beauty.

Below are the 3 main contributors that rob our health and ruin our appearance.

1. Toxicity—Toxic chemicals are in everything: food, air, water, and most products we put on our hair, lips or skin. Toxic overload, nutritionally void diets, and improper gut bacteria are the 3 most common causes of accelerated aging and disease. However, toxic overload may be the leading cause of accelerated aging and disease. This is one factor that causes accelerated aging. When cellular toxicity builds up, cellular DNA is damaged, affecting the skin. This also leads to poorly functioning organs, which in turn leads to disease. I am referring to both internal and external toxins or waste products. External toxins can include heavy metals such as lead, mercury, aluminum, and cadmium. These are all highly damaging to your cells and organs and can lead to rapid aging and disease and death.

Other toxins can include bacterial toxins such as endo- and

neurotoxins, released by numerous bacterial organisms. One such example is the toxins released by the Lyme borrelia bacteria, which often lead to severe organ and nerve damage. These toxins lead to many of the serious symptoms and signs of this disease. Mold mycotoxins are also particularly dangerous and can lead to a wide range of health issues and diseases.

Toxins can and do lead to DNA damage which then leads to improper cellular division which is the basis of all diseases, including cancer. No matter how well you live your life in other areas, if you fail to remove toxins from your body on a regular basis you will age rapidly, get sick, and gain weight.

There is no doubt that toxins are the leading factor of premature aging. High levels of toxins in the body cause inflammation and are a major cause of heart disease, cancer, auto-immune diseases, diabetes, and more. Your body reacts to foreign invaders, introduced from the food we eat, the water we drink, and the products we rub on our skin, by producing an inflammatory response using numerous immune cells. These cells include natural killer cells, cytotoxic T cells and B cell antibodies. If the immune response is not controlled and is ongoing, this can and does lead to damage to various organs. Examples of immune-related disease are Hashimoto's thyroid disease, Crohn's disease, arthritis, SLE, and even diabetes.

Prescription drugs are also a leading cause of toxin overload. Nearly 70% of Americans are taking at least one prescription drug and more than half take two, Mayo Clinic and Olmsted Medical Center researchers say. This study found that antibiotics, antidepressants, and opioids are most commonly prescribed.

America has been called a pill-popping society. Unfortunately, the statistics bear this out. Nearly 50% of all American adults regularly take at least one prescription drug, and 20% take three or more.

Our increasing reliance on prescription medications has contributed to the growing problem of nutrient depletion. The truth is that nearly every medication, including over-the-counter drugs, depletes your body of specific, vital nutrients. This is especially concerning when you consider that most Americans are already suffering from nutrient depletion.

Certain medications can bind with nutrients and inhibit their absorption. For example, acid-reducing drugs can impact the absorption of vitamin B12 while antibiotics can destroy "good" bacteria in the digestive system that play a role in the digestion and absorption of vitamins and minerals. On the other hand, some nutrient-rich foods and dietary supplements can interfere with the effectiveness of medications. Before you take any medication or supplement, talk to your doctor or a healthcare professional to discuss possible interactions and what steps you can take to ensure your body is effectively obtaining and absorbing important nutrients.

Additionally, many of the conditions physicians see often stem from nutrient deficiency or depletion. The good news is that once you are armed with information found in this book, and the desire to begin consuming nutrient-rich fruits and vegetables as well as the right supplements, you can avoid the side effects of nutrient depletion. Even better, you may be able to control and prevent chronic diseases such as diabetes, cardiovascular disease, and osteoporosis.

To understand the role various medications play in causing nutrient depletion, we must first look at the variety of nutrient-depleting mechanisms in the pharmacy.

Many drugs, such as Ritalin (methylphenidate) and Adderall, are prescribed for attention deficit disorder (ADD). These drugs often suppress appetite which, in turn, decreases the intake of essential nutrients. Some anti-depressants also have this appetite-reducing effect.

Certain medications reduce the absorption of specific nutrients into the gastrointestinal tract by binding to them before they're absorbed into the bloodstream. The antibiotic tetracycline, for example, can block absorption by binding with minerals such as calcium, magnesium, iron, and zinc in the GI tract. Weight loss drugs and cholesterol-lowering medicines similarly bind to fats, preventing them from being absorbed. Drugs that treat acid reflux or heartburn raise pH levels in the upper GI tract, which reduces absorption of vitamins and minerals. This is especially problematic for the elderly, who are often already low in stomach acid.

On the flip side, some drugs can deplete nutrition intake by increasing the desire for unhealthy foods, such as refined carbohydrates. Many neuroleptics (anti-psychotic drugs) and some antidepressants cause insulin resistance or metabolic syndrome, with results in blood sugar swings. This often causes cravings that lead to consumption of simple carbohydrates, such as sugar, bread and pasta. Steroid-related drugs, including those taken via inhaler, often create a similar type of craving. Both drugs and parasites have the ability to alter signals in the brain that cause you to crave processed and fast foods.

Nutrients are essential to the metabolic activities of every organ, bone, and cell in the body. They're used up in the process and need to be replaced by eating fruits and vegetables and/or supplements. Some drugs deplete nutrients by speeding up this metabolic rate. These drugs include antibiotics (including penicillin and gentamicin) and steroids such as prednisone and colchicine.

Other drugs block the nutrient's effects at the cellular level. In addition to the effects they have on enzymes or receptors, medications can influence enzymes or receptors that help process essential nutrients. For example, widely prescribed statin drugs block the activity of HMG-CoA, an enzyme that's required to manufacture cholesterol in the body. This action also depletes the body of coenzyme Q10 (CoQ10), which requires HMG-CoA for its production. This has a serious negative impact on muscle and heart health.

Drugs also can increase the loss of nutrients through the urinary system. Any drug that does this can drain the body's levels of water-soluble nutrients, including vitamins and minerals, such as magnesium and potassium. The major offenders are medications to treat hypertension, particularly the diuretics that reduce blood pressure by increasing the volume of water flushed out of the body.

Unfortunately, older people are more susceptible to the side effects of drugs for several reasons:

- As you age, the amount of water in the body decreases, and fat tissue increases. In older people, drugs that dissolve in water reach higher toxic concentrations, because there is less water to dilute them. Drugs that dissolve in fat accumulate more in older adults, because there is more fat tissue to store them.
- As we age, the kidneys are less able to excrete drugs into urine, and the liver is less able to break down many drugs. Thus, drugs are less readily removed from the body.
- Older people usually take more drugs and have more disorders.
- People who take more drugs have a higher risk of drug interactions.
- Fewer studies today are done to help identify appropriate doses of drugs for older people.
- Older people are more likely to have chronic medical disorders that may be negatively affected by drugs or affect how the drugs work.

Because of these age-related changes, many drugs stay in an older person's body much longer, prolonging the drug's effect and increasing the risk of side effects. Therefore, older people often need to drink more water, consume more nutrient-rich foods in their diets, and take smaller doses of certain drugs, or perhaps fewer daily doses. For example, digoxin, a drug sometimes used to treat certain heart disorders, dissolves in water and is eliminated by the kidneys. Because the amount of water in the body decreases and the kidneys function less efficiently as people age, digoxin concentrations in the body may increase, resulting in a greater risk of side effects, such as nausea or abnormal heart rhythms.

Older people are also more sensitive to the effects of many drugs. For example, older people tend to become sleepier and are more likely to become confused when using anti-anxiety drugs or sleep aids to treat insomnia. Some drugs that lower blood pressure tend to lower blood pressure more dramatically in older people, which can lead to side effects such as dizziness, light-headedness, and falls.

As you age, your body becomes less efficient at extracting and absorbing nutrients from the foods you eat, or supplements you take. Eating or juicing more nutrient-dense foods, such as richly colored fruits and vegetables, can help improve your health and overall appearance. Remember the saying, *you are what you eat?* Make it your mission to stop and think, "Is the food I'm eating giving me what I need to look and feel my best?" When you choose a variety of colorful fruits and veggies, whole grains, and lean proteins, you'll feel vibrant and look radiant from the inside out.

In summary, prescription drugs, with all of the side effects that accompany them, have become a part of getting older that people often don't think much about. As you're learning, however, many medications have side effects that can make you feel older, faster! Don't assume that there aren't alternatives to prescription drugs, as some doctors and pharmaceuticals ads would have you believe. It's worth at least seeking out other means to improve your health and symptoms before relying on a drug to do so.

Alcohol consumption also affects nutrient absorption. Alcohol may encourage the swift breakdown of pills and capsules before they reach the small intestine where absorption occurs. It can also interfere with normal digestion by damaging cells in the stomach and intestine interfering with the release of important digestive enzymes. Alcohol also acts as a diuretic, which promotes excretion of stored minerals such as calcium and magnesium. Reduce alcohol's negative impact on nutrient absorption by avoiding it within four hours of juicing.

Alcohol also dehydrates your body generally. Drinking too much is also thought to deprive the skin of vital vitamins and nutrients. Not only does alcohol not offer any nutritional value, it can adversely affect your vitamin and mineral levels by causing depletion in healthy nutrients that aid in carrying oxygen throughout your body. More importantly, alcohol can have a huge negative impact on your vitamin A, B3, and C levels, all of which are very important antioxidants for your skin and vital in the regeneration of new cells.

Facial flushing is probably the most common skin sign of drinking alcohol as intake causes the blood vessels in the skin to dilate even with moderate intake, increasing blood flow. Over time, dilation of blood vessels can become permanent, leading to the formation *ectasia* (i.e. spider veins). These affect mainly the face, chest, abdomen, arms, and hands. The permanent dilation can be caused by not only the direct effect alcohol has on blood vessels, but is in some cases due to liver damage from long-term overindulgence. Furthermore, damage to these small blood vessels can cause them to be leaky, allowing for fluid to enter soft tissue like the skin, giving a puffy, swollen appearance.

Alcohol consumption can also impair the immune system, in addition to disrupting the barrier function of the skin. Both bacterial and fungal skin infections are common in those who drink frequently and excessively. There is some evidence suggesting this immune suppression can also increase the risk of skin cancer, though associated risky behaviors such as smoking and unprotected sun exposure may be compounding factors.

Over time, drinking heavily can have other, more permanent effects on your skin. Rosacea, a skin disorder that starts with a tendency to blush and flush easily and can eventually lead to facial disfigurement, is linked to alcohol.

Similar to alcohol, caffeine can promote excretion of vitamins and minerals. In excessive amounts, tannins (a type of plant compound) found in caffeine can also inhibit the absorption of calcium, iron, magnesium and B-vitamins. Limit your consumption of caffeine to one or two cups of coffee or tea per day, between meals, or drink decaffeinated or caffeine-free beverages.

Our bodies are coated and crusted with years of toxic buildup that coats our digestive systems and organs. Unless you detoxify the body first, you will waste your time and money by juicing and/ or eating raw fresh vitamin- and mineral-rich foods.

2. **Chronic Malnutrition**—The number two root cause of premature aging and disease can be traced back to lack of nutrition.

Chronic malnutrition is a persistent lack of access to necessary vitamins and minerals, leading to health problems and accelerated aging. People who are malnourished tend to develop more slowly, and may remain physically small even as adults. In addition, they can exhibit telltale signs of poor nutrition, such as losing their hair, having flaky or brittle fingernails, and being physically weak and tired. In addition, chronic malnutrition exposes people to the risk of cognitive disabilities caused by not getting enough to eat to maintain brain health.

Nutrition is not simply about the quantity of food people consume, but also the quality. People with chronic malnutrition are sometimes overweight as a result of their diets, but they are still not receiving the balance of vitamins and nutrients they need to survive.

Making matters worse, by the time produce is delivered to a grocery store it's often four to six days old, or picked prematurely, and thus lacking vitamins, minerals, and enzymes. Produce purchased today in markets have already lost up to 50% of its original nutritional value before you even put it in your fridge. Further studies show that if you cook food it kills most, if not all nutritional value. So even if you eat lots of cooked fruits and vegetables, you are only getting a fraction of the recommended daily allowance of vitamins, minerals and enzymes. A new government report shows only about 1 out of 10 Americans eats enough fruits and vegetables. Part of the problem might be that people are not educated on what is required for proper nutrition and find it daunting to eat the daily recommendation of fruits and vegetables.

3. **Imbalance of Gut Bacteria**—Last but not least, bad gut bacteria, also known as candida or yeast overgrowth, can affect your inability to lose weight, your health and appearance significantly. There are over 100 trillion micro-organisms or bacteria in your digestive tract, outnumbering the cells in your entire body. Your gut is so packed with bacteria that over half of your stool is not from what you ate, but from discarded bacteria and *their* waste. And as fast as the bad bacteria are discarded, they are replaced just as quickly.

If you want to restore your health and appearance, you must get your gut in balance. The gut literally affects the entire body. Over 70% of immune-related cells come from your gut. Generally speaking, if you have frequent digestive symptoms and/or discomfort, you likely have a problem with the balance of bacteria in the gut. What is often overlooked, however, is that many other ongoing health and appearance problems can be related directly to unhealthy digestive micro flora as well.

So why is it that rebalancing the bacteria in your gut affects your appearance and other areas of the body? The answer lies in the fact that the intestinal tract contains more chemicals detection and signaling molecules than any other organ in the body, and those molecules affect many aspects of your mood, health, and appearance. Most health-related issues are due to an overgrowth of pathogenic bacteria (bad bacteria), like *candida*, in the gut. The same issues may also result from weaknesses in the gut membrane, and a whole host of digestive-related issues and chronic diseases that can lead to needing to take medication that often kills good bacteria.

3. Parasites—Parasitic infestations are a serious issue, and several sources estimate that 85% of Americans have parasites. Parasites are typically picked up through food and water, and infection can lead to serious health problems. Unfortunately, most doctors are not trained to treat parasites infestations. Often symptoms go unnoticed or misdiagnosed. American doctors often treat the symptoms of parasites. It is only when parasites are **visually** seen that doctors will suspect them. By that time, however, they have already caused great damage to the body. Many species of parasites are so small they can virtually travel anywhere in the body via the bloodstream, so small they may never be seen at all.

Common Parasites

- **Round worms:** Living in the stomach and intestines, these worms enter the body through undercooked and contaminated food. Unfortunately, the manure used in organic farming can easily be contaminated with worms.

Therefore, it is recommended to thoroughly wash your produce, and *always* wash your hands after having contact with raw meats, poultry, and fish, and after handing your pets.

- **Tape worms:** These worms enter the body through under-cooled beef, fish or pork. They live in the lower intestinal tract. Use gloves and wash thoroughly after preparing meat for consumption to prevent them.

- **Pin worms:** Living inside the intestinal tract and lungs, these small white worms come out at night to lay eggs around the anus. The eggs hatch, and then the young worms reenter through the anus. If the person scratches during his sleep, the eggs get under the fingernails and spread to wherever the person touches. It is believed that they are small and lightweight enough to become airborne, leading people to inhale them. This is how they are purported to arrive inside the lungs.

- **Hook worms and thread worms:** These can be found in contaminated drinking water, or they can enter directly through the soles of bare feet, even without open wounds. Always wear shoes when walking outside. These worms are unique because they have a lifespan of several years, and the eggs can incubate for up to ten years.

Symptoms of Parasite Infection

- Repeated diarrhea or constipation
- Chronic or unexplained nausea, often accompanied by vomiting
- Fatigue and weakness
- Intestinal cramping

- Unexplained dizziness
- Foul-smelling gas
- Indigestion
- Bloating
- Multiple food allergies
- Loss of appetite
- Itching around the anus, especially at night
- Difficulty sleeping
- Difficulty maintaining a healthy weight (over or under-weight)
- Itching on the soles of the feet, often accompanied by a rash
- Coughing blood (severe cases)
- Palpitations (hook worms)
- Anemia
- Facial swelling around the eyes (round worms)
- Wheezing and coughing, followed by vomiting, stomach pain, and bloating (suggesting round worms or thread worms)
- Itching or tingling sensations on the scalp

CHAPTER 3

CHEMICALS AND TOXINS

Over the last one hundred years, over seventy-five thousand chemicals have been invented and are currently in use today. They are all around us. According to a recent documentary "The Human Experiment" over forty-two billion (yes, billion) pounds of chemicals enter American commerce every single day. In the last fifty years, chemical use and consumption has increased 2000%. It's no surprise that disease and cancer have increased right alongside this significant increase in chemical use. The foods we eat, water we drink, plastic bottles we use, toothpaste, sun screens, makeup, beauty lotions, carpets, curtains, air fresheners, cleaning products, deodorants, etc. — all of these and tens of thousands more contain chemicals.

Toxic exposure from air pollutants, herbicides, pesticides, and personal care and household chemicals result in the accumulation of free radicals in our bodies. These compound over the years and begin an inflammatory process, and ultimately cause oxidative stress. In addition, simply by processing the energy from our food, our bodies are actually producing hundreds of millions of free radicals at any given time. We are constantly being bombarded with free radicals that end up causing oxidative stress, inflammation, aging, and disease.

The best thing we can do aside from getting sleep, water, and proper nutrition, is to limit our exposure. In this book you will learn the truth about chemicals hidden in products, foods and water. You will learn how they affect the body and how to eliminate them.

Think you're not toxic? Feel that you're healthy? Drink plenty of water? Eat a well balanced diet? Think again. If you suffer from one of these symptoms, your body is toxic and causing you to age prematurely.

1. Do you feel fatigued most of the time?
2. Does your weight fluctuate?
3. Do you have bad breath?
4. Do you suffer from constipation?
5. Are you smell- or scent-sensitive?
6. Do you have muscle ache and pains?
7. Do you have acne or red blotchy skin?
8. Do you have mood swings?
9. Irritable bowels?
10. Headaches?

Virtually every non-organic food we eat or product we use is either a chemical or has been treated with chemicals, or genetically modified, which overwhelms our bodies with chemicals and makes it impossible to completely eliminate all the waste and toxins we take in on a daily basis. The good news is that our bodies are designed to remove toxins, heal, and regenerate themselves. However, due to the overwhelming abundance of toxic chemicals we are exposed to as well as the lack of proper hydration and nutrition, our bodies don't have a chance to efficiently process all the toxins it takes in on any given day. Instead they store these toxins, which causes the body to become less efficient and accelerates the aging process.

The good news is that our bodies are very resilient—to a point. The body starts taking measures to dilute the toxins by either retaining water and/or producing fat cells, where these toxins can be stored with the hope of eliminating them the next day. But the truth of the matter is it never does get a chance to do so, and keeps building up day in, day out, until disease sets in—or death.

A bigger problem is human ignorance. You might think, "If

these foods and products treated with chemicals that we eat and use daily are being sold on store shelves, surely they must be safe for consumption or use." But this is the biggest misconception of all. Most, if not all, chemically treated foods and products are not even required by law to be tested for human consumption or safety. In fact, only a tiny percentage of chemicals are regulated. How could this be, you ask? What about the Toxic Substances Control Act (TSCA), a 1976 law that protects humans and the environment from toxic industrial chemicals? Well, pesticides, drugs, and cosmetics are all regulated under different laws, which has created so many hoops for regulators to jump through that it has often rendered them powerless. That's one rationale that the Government Accountability Office, Congress's nonpartisan watchdog arm, has cited in repeatedly calling toxic chemical regulation a huge problem.

Chemical companies are free to create a chemical that may be toxic for human consumption or use. Even if the chemical causes health issues or death, the accountability blame game is often played by multi-billion dollar companies that consider lawsuits, research, and human casualties a cost of doing business. Such companies have systems in place to defer blame and keep their poisonous chemicals in use, despite overwhelming evidence that their chemical causes disease and death. In fact, it's so common a practice to defend toxic chemicals' harmful effects on humans and animals that the industrial companies that produce them have a playbook strategy they use borrowed from the tobacco and drug companies called "The Four Dog Defense."

The Four Dog Defense

1. My dog does not bite–

This first line of defense uses arguments that the studies

conducted show the dangers of the chemical are from sources that are not qualified or are biased. For example the chemical company will produce studies that show there's no problem using their chemical or there isn't enough evidence or proof.

2. My dog does bite, but it didn't bite you–

Once there is enough proof that people are getting sick and/or evidence that their chemical causes harm to humans and animals, the following defense is used. Ok, our chemical may be harmful, but no one is exposed to it or comes into direct contact with it. Or they defer, and demand you prove that their chemical got into your body.

3. My dog bit you but it did not hurt you–

This line of defense comes in when there is overwhelming evidence that their chemical may be out there, in people, pets, wildlife and/or the environment and is causing harm. They make the argument that you would have to consume or be exposed to an unrealistic amount of their chemical to make your sick, or the animal studies that were conducted don't mean anything for humans or the environment.

4. My dog bit you, but it wasn't my fault.

This line of defense is when there is undeniable evidence that their chemical causes disease or death in humans and affecting the environment. They argue it's not their fault people consume it. It's the consumer's choice to use their product. We didn't force them to use it. Alternatively, it's because those people also had bad eating habits, did not exercise, or took other drugs or alcohol that might have caused the death or disease. At this point they are forced to put warning labels on the product, but allowed to keep producing and selling their deadly chemical.

As you can see by this cold, never-my-fault, blame-deflecting defensive strategy, which proves how little value they place on human life when it comes to protecting their profits, it's no surprise why these cancer-causing chemicals remain in use. All these companies have to do once the evidence becomes overwhelming is put a warning label on their dangerous, often deadly chemicals. That's it. Then business continues as usual.

What's more disturbing is the misconception that the food we eat and products we use are safe, and the lack of motivation to learn what's in them—and our government's reactive approach to chemical safety and controls.

Even more alarming is a 2009 study from Scientific American done on newborn babies, that found trace elements of 232 synthetic chemicals in umbilical cord blood from ten different ethnic groups born in 2009, in different parts of the United States. These newborn babies were tested before they took their first meal or breath. The study was initially looking for a chemical called Bisphenal A (BPA), a plastic component and synthetic estrogen widely used in food and plastic drink storage containers. Sadly, and not surprisingly, BPA turned up in 9 of the 10 umbilical cord blood samples tested. Even worse is the whole host of new chemicals the study detected in the babies' umbilical cord blood.

The study focused on contaminates from exposure to consumer products and the commercial chemicals omnipresent on supermarket shelves. The study showed a significant failure on Congress's part, and on that of the government agencies charged with protecting human health. The study strongly suggests that the health of all children is threatened by trace amounts of hundreds of synthetic chemicals coursing though their bodies.

Since the chemical revolution, we have seen childhood diseases rise significantly.

- Childhood brain cancer up 38%

- Asthma up 80%
- Leukemia in children 74%
- Early-onset puberty 55%
- ADHD 53%
- Genital deformities in baby boys 122%
- Life-threatening birth defects 100%

Below are just a <u>fraction</u> of the chemicals they found in their study.

Acrylamides—Acrylamide is a chemical used primarily for the production of paper, dyes, and plastics, and in the treatment of drinking water and wastewater, including sewage. It is also found in consumer products such as caulking, food packaging, and some adhesives. Trace amounts of acrylamide generally remain in these products. Researchers in Europe and the United States have also found acrylamide in certain foods, with potato chips and french fries containing the highest levels. The World Health Organization and the Food and Agriculture Organization of the United Nations stated that the levels of acrylamide in foods pose a "major concern" and more research is needed to determine the risk of dietary acrylamide exposure [2].

Recombinant Bovine Growth Hormone (RBGH)—RBGH and Rbst—rBGH (recombinant Bovine Growth Hormone) and rBST (recombinant bovine somatotropin) are two genetically engineered, potent variants of the natural growth hormone produced by cows. Manufactured by Monsanto, it is sold to dairy farmers under the trade name POSILAC. Injections of this hormone forces cows to increase their milk production by about 10%. Monsanto has stated that about one third of dairy cows are in herds where the hormone is used.

Dr. Samuel S. Epstein, Professor Emeritus of environmental medicine at the University of Illinois at Chicago School of Public

Health and world renowned author, published his book, "What's in Your Milk?" which was a powerful exposure of the dangers of Monsanto's genetically-engineered (rBGH*) milk, and the company's no-holds-barred conspiracy to suppress this information.

Monsanto, supported by the Food and Drug Administration (FDA), insists that rBGH milk is indistinguishable from natural milk and that it is safe for consumers. This is, however, blatantly false. RBGH makes cows sick. Monsanto has been forced to admit to about twenty toxic effects, including mastitis, on its Posilac label.

*rBGH milk is contaminated by pus, due to the mastitis commonly induced by rBGH, and antibiotics used to treat the mastitis.

*rBGH milk is chemically and nutritionally different than natural milk. *Milk from cows injected with rBGH is contaminated with the hormone, traces of which are absorbed through the gut into the blood. *rBGH milk is supercharged with high levels of a natural growth factor (IGF-1) which is readily absorbed through the gut. *Excess levels of IGF-1 have been identified as a cause of breast, colon, and prostate cancers. IGF-1 blocks natural defense mechanisms against early submicroscopic cancers. *rBGH enriches Monsanto while posing dangers, without any benefits, to consumers, especially in view of the current national surplus of milk.

Pyrethroids—Pyrethrins and pyrethroids are insecticides included in over 3,500 registered products, many of which are used widely in and around households, including on pets, for the purpose of mosquito control and in agriculture. The use of pyrethrins and pyrethroids has increased during the past decade with the declining use of organophosphate pesticides, which are more acutely toxic to birds and mammals than the pyrethroids. This change to less acutely toxic pesticides, while beneficial, has introduced certain new issues. For example, residential uses of pyrethrins and pyrethroids may result in urban runoff, exposing aquatic life to harmful levels in water and sediment.

Heavy metals—The term heavy metal refers to any metallic chemical element that has a relatively high density and is toxic or poisonous at low concentrations. Examples of heavy metal include mercury (Hg), cadmium (Cd), arsenic (As), chromium (Cr), thallium (Tl) and lead (Pb). As trace elements, some heavy metals are essential to maintain the metabolism of the human body. However, at higher concentrations they can lead to poisoning. Heavy metal poisoning could result, for instance, from water contamination (e.g. lead pipes), high ambient air concentrations near emission sources, or intake via the food chain.

Heavy metals are dangerous because they tend to increase in concentration in a biological organism over time, compared to the chemical's concentration in the environment. Compounds accumulate in living things any time they are taken up and stored faster than they are broken down (metabolized) or excreted.

Aromatic Hydrocarbons—Various substances and industrial processes, surrogates of exposure to polycyclic aromatic hydrocarbons (PAHs), are currently classified as human carcinogens. Studies showed direct evidence of the carcinogenic effects of PAHs in occupationally exposed subjects. Risks of lung and bladder cancer were dose dependent when PAHs were measured quantitatively and truly nonexposed groups were chosen for comparison. These new findings suggest that the current threshold limit value of 0.2 mg/m3 of benzene soluble matter (which indicates PAH exposure) is unacceptable because, after forty years of exposure, it involves a relative risk of 1.2-1.4 for lung cancer and 2.2 for bladder cancer.

Polybrominated Diphenyl Ethers—An increased incidence of thyroid cancer has been reported in many parts of the world, including the United States, during the past several decades. Recently emerging evidence has demonstrated that polyhalogenated aromatic hydrocarbons (PHAHs), particularly polybrominated diphenyl ethers (PBDEs), cause thyroid dysfunction. However, few studies have been conducted to test whether exposure to PBDEs and other PHAHs increases the risk of thyroid cancer. Elevated exposure to PHAHs, particularly PBDEs, increases the risk of thyroid cancer and may explain part of the increase in incidences of thyroid cancer during the past several decades. In addition, genetic and epigenetic variations in metabolic pathway genes may alter the expression and function of metabolic enzymes which are involved in the metabolism of endogenous thyroid hormones and the detoxification of PBDEs and other PHAHs. Such variation may result in different individual susceptibilities to PBDEs and other PHAHs, and the subsequent development of thyroid cancer.

Benzophenone from Sunblock—Some of the chemical ingredients in sunscreens are totally prohibited by the FDA. Other synthetic chemicals may be included among the FDA-prescribed and regulated chemical substances but are harmful only if used in levels beyond what is regulated. However, hazard warnings are still up, since their toxic effects will depend on the consumer's frequency of application or use. There are in fact thousands of chemical substances and derivatives used in different industries, and more than a hundred of them have been found as cancer-causing ingredients in sunscreens.

Per Fluorocarbons (PFCs)—Dr. Shoreh Ershadi, director of the Anti-Aging Institute of California, wants to bring to the attention of menopausal women that now there may be a link between early menopause and exposure to common PFCs or per fluorocarbons which inhibit hormone functioning. PFCs are used in a wide range of products, including non-stick cookware, personal care products, packaging, and furniture treatment chemical residues. PFCs can also be found in water, animals, soil, plants, and people.

Here are just a few of the toxic reasons why you should be reading personal care ingredient labels just as closely as you read those on the foods we eat. "Fragrance" as an ingredient often hides any number of chemicals in a personal care product. Many fragrances are toxic. Some of these fragrances may be phthalates, which can act as obesogens (cause obesity) and may disrupt normal endocrine function, including reproductive health. Phthalates may cause developmental defects and delays.

Talc, another common ingredient, is a known carcinogen. It is used to absorb moisture and provide a hint of sparkle. It is found in eye shadow, blush, baby powder, deodorant and soap. Talc is directly linked to ovarian cancer and acts similarly to asbestos when inhaled, and may lead to lung tumors.

Your skin is the largest organ in the human body, and it is permeable. Skin does not provide the defenses and toxic waste disposal that your body's digestive system does. Toxins are absorbed directly from the skin into your fat cells, and often into the blood stream. People who are trying to look younger by using lotions filled with toxic chemicals will see the opposite effect in the long run!

Pesticides and Herbicides

The levels of pesticides (bug killing chemicals) and herbicides (weed killing chemicals) in our food supply are also on the rise, contributing significantly to our daily toxic load. While organic foods may be a bit more expensive, our support of organic farming efforts will help mitigate costs, as well as promote sustainable, eco-friendly farming. Though many argue the value of organic foods, certainly anyone concerned with limiting their overall exposures to chemical pollutants will agree it is worth a few extra dollars per day to not only do that, but support the efforts of people who are against the big agrochemical corporations ruining our rainforests and poisoning our food supply in the name of profit.

Chlorinated Pesticides

Chlorinated pesticides are nerve agents used in agriculture as pesticides to kill insects. These toxic chemicals were designed to attack the nervous system of pests, which lead to overstimulation of the nerves and eventually death. The most well-known chlorinated pesticide is DDT (dichlorodiphenyltrichloroethane).

DDT is a colorless, crystalline, tasteless and almost odorless organochloride known for its insecticidal properties. Most chlorinated pesticides have been banned for use in the United States since the 1980s. However, some of these chemicals are still in use in other parts of the world and, as fat-soluble toxins, are imported to the United States for consumption. These chemicals have been found in fatty tissue of animals and humans.

Human exposure occurs mainly through our diet, primarily from high fat foods such as, meat, poultry, dairy products, and fish, and non-organic leafy and root vegetables. Other sources of exposure are from contaminated dust and soil.

Chlorinated pesticides are fat-soluble toxins, which means they are stored in our body fat and in the fat of the animals we consume. Acute toxicity from chlorinated pesticides is rarely seen since they have been banned; however, their persistence in the environment and our bodies can cause a variety of health problems. The effects of these compounds are most often seen in the neurological, immunological, and endocrinological systems, although they can also affect the cardiovascular, respiratory, gastrointestinal, and other systems in the body.

Fruits and Vegetables

Non-organic fruits and vegetables often contain chlorinated pesticides due to nutrient absorption from contaminated soil. Farmers spray the produce and water the crops, and the chemicals are absorbed into the plant from the soil as it absorbs water.

Meat

Chlorinated pesticides are stored in fatty tissues. When we consume fatty meats, we are also consuming these toxins. Animals are exposed to pesticides in their natural environment due to groundwater contamination and bioaccumulation. It is recommended to limit fatty meat intake to lower chlorinated pesticide exposure.

Dairy

Due to the fact that chlorinated pesticides are stored in fatty tissues, dairy products also contain these toxins. Animals are exposed to these pesticides in their natural environment due to groundwater contamination and bioaccumulation.

Fish

A number of fresh water fish advisories have been posted in certain US lakes and rivers because of DDT and PCB contamination of trout and other fish.

Fruit

Fruit may be contaminated with pesticides that are used either directly or by chemical residues that attach to the fruit via dust particles in the environment. Again, it's my recommendation to buy organic.

Organophosphate pesticides

Similar to the chemical warfare agents produced during World War II, organophosphates (OPs) are some of the most common and most toxic insecticides used today, adversely affecting the human nervous system even at low levels of exposure.

Research shows a range of neurotoxin developmental problems associated with prenatal and early childhood exposure:

- Impaired short-term memory and mental development
- Increased reaction time & abnormal reflexes
- Mental & emotional problems (adolescent exposure)

Fruits and vegetables that are commonly eaten by children, including peaches, apples, grapes, green beans, and pears, are among the foods most commonly contaminated with organophosphates. (Source: WhatsOnMyFood.org) Developing children are the most susceptible to chemical pesticides. They can be exposed through the air, food, dust, soil, and even pets. Children of farm workers and children in agricultural areas are among the most exposed to OPs, although urban children are also at risk.

Among the most acutely toxic pesticides, most organophosphates are classified by the U.S. Environmental Protection Agency as highly or moderately toxic. They interfere with the nervous system by inhibiting an enzyme called acetylcholinesterase. Under normal conditions, acetylcholinesterase controls nerve impulses by sending chemical signals to halt the nerve impulse at the appropriate time. When organophosphates impede this process, the nervous system becomes severely over-stimulated, resulting in immediate neurological dysfunction. Symptoms of acute exposure include nausea, headaches, twitching, trembling, excessive salivation, tearing, inability to breathe, convulsions, and, at higher doses, death.

Longer term, lower dose exposure to organophosphate pesticides is linked to a number of health problems:

- Developmental Effects: Organophosphates interfere with healthy neurodevelopment, leading to behavioral problems and lower cognitive function. Children exposed to this type of pesticides are more likely to develop ADHD, a recent study shows.

- Reproductive Effects: As endocrine disrupters, organophosphates have a significant impact on the human reproductive system. The presence of OP metabolites in the body is associated with reduced levels of testosterone and other sex hormones. Exposure to OPs may have an adverse effect on male fertility.

- Cancer: Although most OPs are not considered carcinogenic, the CDC reports that several studies link organophosphate exposure to leukemia and lymphoma. The U.S. EPA also classifies the Opdiclorvos as a "probable human carcinogen."

- Parkinson's Disease: Since OPs affect the brain; it's not surprising that they have been linked to neurological disorders. Living near application sites of diazinon, chlorpyrifos, or dimethoate has been found to increase the risk of Parkinson's disease.

Chemical companies that produce these toxic chemicals assure us that they are safe for human consumption. Albeit at low doses, several reports from chemical companies claim the chemicals are safe. However, young children and older adults are more susceptible to the side effects.

Although all these chemicals were found in unborn babies blood albeit at trace amounts. The real problem is that our bodies don't get a chance to eliminate these toxins due to toxic overload and starts storing these harmful toxins. Unless the kidneys and liver can remove them, they can reach dangerous levels that cause disease, and cause the cells and skin to age prematurely.

CHAPTER 4

HOW TO REMOVE
AGE-ROBBING TOXINS

Every day, we are exposed to harmful chemicals and toxins that accelerate aging and disease, including bisphenol-A (BPA), phthalates, PFOA, formaldehyde, PDBEs, and heavy metals. They can be found in everything, from beauty products to cookware, from the food we eat to the air we breathe. It's critical that you reduce your exposure to these age robbing toxins by choosing organic non-processed foods and non-toxic products whenever possible, and make sure your home and work environments are properly ventilated. We're also bombarded with toxins from processed, fried foods, non-organic foods, alcohol, stimulants, medications, and much more. These toxins accumulate over time and damage our DNA, create inflammation, and impair critical biological functions.

Reduce your exposure by choosing all-natural foods and non-toxic products whenever possible, and make sure your home and work environments are properly ventilated. Have yourself tested (or try an elimination diet) if you feel you may be sensitive to gluten, dairy, eggs, or other allergenic foods that can increase the permeability of your digestive tract, allowing toxins to enter your circulation.

A healthy detoxification program should always begin gradually. With so many methods available, it can be difficult to find a starting point. With that in mind, I would like to share some of my top-recommended steps—through my experience—for safe and effective detoxification.

Before you start your *Juice Your Way Back 10 Years* challenge, you must first get your body back to a restorative, non-toxic state.

You should start slowly, day by day, week by week, and month by month. Once I learned all the dangers of chemical toxins, it took me some time to remove most toxins from my food, water, and the products I ate and used daily. Notice that I used the words "most toxins," as it's virtually impossible to remove all toxins that enter the body. By following the steps below, and letting the body heal and restore balance, you will notice a significant difference in your skin, energy, health, and appearance.

Don't get overwhelmed, or think you have to be a toxin-free freak. Remember that it's taken you years to build up your current high levels of toxic chemicals and waste in your body, and that it will take sometime to identify and eliminate these age-robbing toxins completely from your body and life.

In order to maximize your goals of looking and feeling younger, you <u>must</u> make drastic changes in the things you are now doing— without exception. Your life, health, and appearance depend upon it. They say insanity is doing the same thing and expecting different results, and unless you make immediate changes in your life, your health and pre-mature aging will drastically accelerate and deteriorate.

The body has two major organs whose job it is to eliminate and neutralize toxins. One is the liver, and the other is the kidneys. However, if you body is overloaded with toxins, dehydrated, and undernourished, these organs may not be running at optimal performance due to the damage done from processed foods, smoking, prescription medication, and alcohol. Over time, toxins can attach to the linings of your digestive system and harden, causing any vitamins or nutrients you eat, take, or drink to simply pass right though, further exacerbating the problem.

The problem is that the walls of your small intestine, where 90% of all nutrients are absorbed, get covered with toxic mucus and stagnant bile. This leads to poor digestion and non-absorption of nutrients in the small intestines, which fill up with gas, yeast, and parasites. Side effects include bloating, abdominal discomfort, or even pain. Stress can irritate this condition by slowing down the food traffic and creating further toxins, which poison your system by clogging it, making you constipated, tired, and fatigued.

"The intestines can store a vast amount of this partially digested, putrefying matter," claims natural health expert Richard Anderson, N.D., N.M.D. "Some intestines, when autopsied, have weighed up to forty pounds and were distended to a diameter of twelve inches with only a pencil-thin channel through which the feces could move. That forty pounds was due to caked layers of encrusted mucus, mixed with fecal matter, bizarrely resembling hardened blackish-green truck tire rubber, or an old piece of dried rawhide." This waste matter is highly toxic and suppresses your immune system, potentially causing gas, bloating, and constipation, dramatically reducing the assimilation of nutrients, slowing your metabolism, and making you sick.

These toxic poisons include everything from vaccines, non-prescription and prescription drugs, the air we breath, the water in which we shower, bathe, swim, and drink, the chemicals put in our food and on our skin, which are all absorbed and stored in our bodies. This also includes chemical toxins from carpeting, paint, cosmetics, makeup, soaps lotions, toothpaste and sunscreens. They even come from things as simple as nonstick cookware.

The first basic cleanse you need to do is a juice detox cleanse. I will provide the organic ingredients you will need below to juice or blend during your three-to-five-day *Juice Your Way Back* Cleanse© or you can go to our website and order a cleansing program and have organic juice delivered right to your home or office at www. juiceyourwayback.com.

Some of the beneficial results you will notice once you have removed a majority of the toxins in your body may include weight loss and healthier hair, skin, and nails. Your energy levels may go through the roof. Depression, stress, anxiety and fatigue are usually reduced. Food cravings may decrease and you may sense that you are in control of your life, not a slave to sickness and looking older than you should.

Below is a list of things you must do in order to regain your health and restore your glow, energy, and appearance.

Detox and Cleanse

When was the last time you cleansed, went on a toxin-free diet, had a colonic, or did a one-to-three-day juice fast? From the time you were born until now, your body has been collecting and storing toxins, causing your organs and absorption of nutrients and toxin elimination to be less efficient. It is imperative to eliminate as many toxins as possible from the foods you eat, the water you drink, and the products you use for a minimum of ten to twenty days before you start the *Juice Your Way Back* Challenge.

Otherwise, you are wasting your money and time. What's the point if you start to eat healthy and juice nutrient-dense fruits and vegetables, when your digestive organs are coated with toxic matter that prevents their absorption? Our bodies are programmed to heal, eliminate, and regenerate. With your help, your organs and digestive processes will improve significantly, and aid in the speed and success of the program.

The detoxifying fruits, vegetables, and herbs below do not come with measurements. Don't get hung up on that. Regularity is what will reverse and restore your health and appearance.

When it comes to cleansing your body of harmful toxins, knowledge and juicing really are the best process to flush the body of toxins. You'll be amazed to learn that many of your favorite fruits, veggies and herbs also cleanse the liver, intestines, kidneys, and skin, eliminating and preventing harmful toxic buildup.

They also help ward off the harmful effects of pollution, food additives, second-hand smoke, and other toxins with delicious fruits, vegetables, nuts, oils, and beans. In working with many clients, I have found that many peoples' tastes are different, so by including a robust list of known detoxification ingredients gives you the power to mix and match ingredients to your specific goals and taste.

Instructions: Blend or juice a minimum of three to five ingredients from the list below in one to two juices or smoothies per day. When juicing, remember you will need a lot of the ingredients to get a glass or two of juice, whereas blending doesn't require as many ingredients. Also, it's a great idea to juice larger amounts of ingredients and then freeze them in ice cube trays, so you can juice and blend faster during the week, without as much prep and clean up. See Chapter 14 for additional benefits of juicing and blending on the go and in less than five minutes. Always consult a health care professional before you start any weight loss or detox system. Consult with your doctor and tell him your plans of detoxing and juicing, especially if you're on any medication.

Detoxifying Fruits and Vegetables

(Always wash all ingredients and choose in-season produce—and organic produce when available. Use our list of what ingredients you must buy organic and those that you don't need to buy organic in chapter seven.

Celery – Blood cleanser with detoxifying properties. Celery seeds contain anti-inflammatory substances.

Kale – Antioxidant compound that cleanses the body; high in fiber that cleanses the intestinal tract.

Green Apple – High in pectin, a fiber that binds to heavy metals and cleanses the intestines.

Water – The most natural way to detox, it promotes good digestion by dissolving toxins.

Lemon – Liver detoxifier that includes high amounts of vitamin C to assist in detoxification.

Beets – Excellent detoxification enzyme veggie, high in iron, antioxidants, and purifies blood and liver.

Blackberries, Raspberries – These berries are high in fiber and antioxidants, which replenish the body and purge toxins.

Blueberries – Clean the liver; contain natural aspirin and antioxidants that help lessen inflammation.

Carrots – Bind to toxins and waste material and remove them from the colon.

Brussels Sprouts – A cruciferous plant high in sulfur which also helps to remove toxins from blood.

Grapefruit – Contains just over seventy milligrams of liver-cleansing glutathione, and lowers cholesterol.

Detoxifying Herbs

Cilantro – Binds to heavy metals, thereby purifying tissues, organs and blood.

Ginger – Considered the best detoxifying herb, a good anti-inflammatory, and contains antioxidants.

Watercress – High in antioxidants, vitamins A and C, and increases detoxification enzymes for cleansing.

Parsley – Eliminates salt build up in kidneys, purging the body of poisons, mercury, cadmium, and lead.

Dandelion Tea – Detoxes the liver, purifies bladder and kidneys and regulates blood sugar.

Mint – Cleans the colon, flushes toxins, prevents build up, and adds a cool kick to your smoothie or juice.

Basil – Cleans the kidneys, removes waste and highly processed foods from our blood stream.

The idea is to ease your body into detoxing and proper nutrition. It's recommended that you juice or blend for only three to ten days and drink lots of water when you wake and when you juice. I understand that this might be a challenge. If you cannot commit to a complete fast, then commit to replacing your first meal of the day with a detoxifying juice blend or for lunch or dinner. Should you eat solid foods, choose all-natural, organic foods or meats. The goal is to flush and remove as many toxins as possible first, then flood your cells with anti-aging regenerative superfoods and micronutrients.

After gently detoxifying your circulation and digestion, you can gradually advance to more thorough detoxification of organs and tissues. For an in-depth detox, I recommend incorporating compounds, herbs, and nutrients such as N-acetyl cysteine, selenium, MSM, alpha-lipoic acid, milk thistle, cilantro, goldenrod, garlic, and dandelion leaf. These natural detoxifying agents have their own affinities for specific organs and systems of the body, and work to eliminate toxins without side effects. They help with reducing parasite growth and also boost energy and provide antioxidant support to combat oxidative stress caused during toxin removal.

By following these relatively simple yet important tips for a successful cleanse, you will quickly feel the benefits of reduced stress and anxiety, decreased inflammation, increased energy, better sleep, and improved health and vitality.

1. Parasitic Cleanse

In order rid your body of all types of parasites, a general parasite cleanse can be extremely helpful. But in order to completely eliminate them, it will also be necessary to consume a wide range of foods and juices to ensure you have killed every type of parasites.

1. **Raw Garlic** – One of the number one ways to kill parasites. This blows away all effective parasite cleanses. Always include garlic. Use organic garlic cloves, in my experience its best to cut them in pill forms and swallow then with your juice or smoothie. It's important to note that cutting and or chewing garlic releases the healing antioxidants called Allicin. Always cut or chew before swallowing. Otherwise you are only getting a fraction of the benefits of this amazing healing plant.

Garlic is rich in manganese, calcium, phosphorus, selenium, and vitamins B6 and C, so it's beneficial for your bones as well as your thyroid and killing parasites. It's thought that much of garlic's therapeutic effect comes from its sulfur-containing compounds, such as allicin, which are also what give it its characteristic smell.

Other health-promoting compounds include:

1.   Reducing inflammation (reduces the risk of osteoarthritis and other disease associated with inflammation)

2.   Boosting immune function (antibacterial, antifungal, antiviral, and anti-parasitic properties)

3.   Improving cardiovascular health and circulation (protects against clotting, retards plaque, improves lipids, and reduces blood pressure.

4.   Toxic to 14 kinds of cancer cells (including brain, lung, breast, gastric, and pancreatic)

2. **Organic Apple Cider Vinegar with the Mothers** – This is one of my favorites, and will keep the stomach free of parasites and will also ensure that you will kill off any larvae or parasite eggs you unintentionally eat with your meals. Aids proper digestion and can cure constipation.

- Can help fight bacterial and fungal infections
- Can relieve join pain
- Balance cholesterol
- Can help heal skin conditions such as acne, age spots, and reduces the appearance of cellulite
- Protects against food poisoning
- Increases stamina
- Boosts metabolism and assists with weight loss
- Prevents bladder stones and urinary tract infections
- Known to be helpful with a host of ailments: constipation, headaches, arthritis, weak bones, indigestion, high cholesterol, diarrhea, eczema, sore eyes, chronic fatigue, mild food poisoning, hair loss, high blood pressure, obesity, etc.

Drink apple cider vinegar daily for best results, ideally fifteen minutes before each meal.

The starting dosage is 1 tablespoon in a big glass of water and you can slowly increase the dosage, a teaspoon at a time over several weeks, to 2 or even 3 tablespoons, if you find the increased dosage beneficial to your health.

Yes it does taste a little sour, but that's a good thing. It's important to train your taste buds to not expect everything to be sweet.

If you really can't handle it at the start, then try it with a drop of stevia sweetener. Using sugar or commercial honey to sweeten it will only feed the parasites and intestinal problems that apple cider vinegar is used to treat.

3. Pumpkin Seeds – Can help to get rid of tapeworms.

4. Pineapple – Contains the enzyme Bromelain, an anti-parasitic superfood. It's been rumored that a three-day pineapple fast will kill tapeworms.

5. Cranberry Juice (unsweetened) or Carrot Juice – Cranberry juice can be diluted in water.

6. Coconut Oil – Contains lauric acid, which is found in coconut products. Coconut oil is half comprised of this saturated fat which, after it is converted by the body, creates a substance that efficiently kills parasites, yeasts, viruses, and pathogenic bacteria in the gut.

7. Fennel Seed Tea – A mild laxative. This can be an irritant to certain types of parasites.

8. Herbs – Cloves, Wormwood, Black Walnut Hull and Husks – These herbs are always incorporated into an effective parasite cleanse, and should be among the ingredients listed in the capsules you take daily from parasite cleanses that can be bought in health food stores. Cloves kill parasite eggs that may linger in the intestinal tract. Black walnut hull and wormwood kill the adult and developmental stages of around 100 different types of parasites. All three are essential.

9. Pungent Spices – Turmeric, cinnamon, nutmeg, cloves, cardamom, chilies, horseradish, and cayenne all make parasites run for cover.

10. Probiotics/Fermented Foods – Some options that can be made at home include sauerkraut (fermented cabbage), however in my experience the best option to balancing out your gut and killing yeast causing parasites is a dual encapsulation probiotic. Most probiotics eaten are killed in the stomach from acid and never make it to your intestines. Probiotics help to replenish good bacteria and kill the bad. For the best probiotic to take visit my website and click on supplements.

I do not recommend choosing one of the anti-parasite formulas that are available in retailers, since they are usually overpriced and formulated at very low concentrations.

Diatomaceous earth is probably the best natural anti-parasitic medication. It is a natural pesticide that does not harm humans or pets. It is believed to kill insects, worms, and parasites by dehydrating them. One tablespoon of diatomaceous earth taken by an adult, once a day for seven days, is believed to be extremely effective for killing all parasites. When it is used on children, bear in mind that height is a better indicator of the size of their G.I. tracts than their weights. Thus, a child who is four feet tall should take 2 teaspoons, and a child who is two feet tall should take 1 teaspoon.

If you take the diatomaceous earth route, then we insist you only buy food grade. Industrial diatomaceous earth is used for swimming pool filters, but it has been chemically treated, so this type is not safe to eat. Try to avoid rubbing it onto your hands, since it will have a drying effect upon the skin. Diatomaceous earth contains heavy metals as part of its mineral content, but it also contains selenium, which allows otherwise accumulative heavy metals to be safely flushed from the body. Therefore, it is not really a health concern despite the trace presence of aluminum and lead. We recommend taking selenium supplements for a week after discontinuing this treatment, to ensure that the body thoroughly neutralizes the metals. Concerned individuals can follow the parasite cleanse with a metal cleanse. My research indicates that diatomaceous earth is the best overall parasite treatment for humans, because it can kill blood-borne parasites as well. When using it, be sure to drink plenty of fluids, because it will dehydrate a person considerably.

Wormwood and black walnut hulls are known to kill adult worms, whilst cloves kill eggs. Some people use this trio for treating parasites, instead of diatomaceous earth. It is recommended that you take 500 mg of wormwood and black walnut hulls, whilst taking 1/2 teaspoon of cloves daily for about fourteen days. The other herbs listed can be used to augment these two core protocols.

As parasites die, they release toxins through their excrement and as they rot. The most common parasites, the worm type, attempt to escape by burrowing deeper into the intestines, which can cause sharp cramps. Even when they're dead, the body is still burdened with the task of flushing them out. This whole process can initially make the person feel sicker than before he began the cleanse, but this is only temporary, and it is a sign that the cleanse is working. It is known as a Herxheimer reaction, when people become sicker as a result of the toxins that are released by dying parasites. While fatigue and grogginess are to be expected, normal life may be continued and diarrhea should not occur. Eat a good, wholesome diet throughout your cleanse to ensure the immune system is at its strongest. After cleansing the body of toxins, you should feel better and have more energy.

CHAPTER 5

HOW TO REVERSE PREMATURE AGING

Below are the necessary steps you must take to ensure that you achieve your goals. If followed diligently, they may allow you to slow down and even reverse the aging process. I promise that, if you follow my steps and practice living an organic toxin-free lifestyle, you can reverse aging, restore your health, and feel and look ten to fifteen years younger. Your daily habits, products you use, and foods you eat can either add or subtract years from your life. Below are steps you must take to ensure that your reach your goals. I am not a medical doctor. It is recommended to consult with your doctor and inform them of what you are doing to ensure there are no conflicts with your current medical regimen. I present this information for educational purposes only. The information below is strictly my opinion and based on research that is currently available.

1. Eliminate All Toxic Chemicals

I'm sure by now you're well aware of the detrimental effects of chemicals and toxins we eat, drink and rub all over our body. If you truly want to restore your youthful glow, speed your metabolism and restore your health, this is a must, and a good habit to develop. It took years for your body to accumulate its current levels of toxins, and the detoxifying process will not happen during a three-day juice cleanse, or by drinking teas or powders or quick-fix potions. It will take months, if not years, to allow your body to balance itself. Start today by only allowing non-toxic foods and products in or on your body. You don't need to be a toxin-free freak, but know that you are helping your body run more efficiently by making changes to your daily life. By doing this day in, day out, and by being committed, you will experience the following benefits over time:

Energy Boost – This is achieved by stopping the influx of toxins by cutting out sugar, caffeine, trans fats, saturated fats, and replacing them with nutrient-dense fresh fruits and vegetables. You'll be getting a natural boost without crashing from junk food and canned sodas.

Weight Loss – This is a side effect of giving the body a rest, and then letting it ramp up again without being bogged down from toxic overload. By eliminating fats, sugars, and processed foods, you will begin to lose weight and look better from the rush of nutrients you get from juicing and/or blending. It's easy to see how a reduction in bad foods and good habits will speed weight loss.

Improved Immunity – When you control and eliminate a large percentage of toxins entering your body, you free up your organs from having to work exclusively on toxin elimination. This helps your body fight off illness easier, because it's not detracted from just trying to manage the toxic load it's under. Once freed up, the body will get back to doing with it does best: keeping you healthy.

Improved Skin – Your skin is the largest organ in the body and often is the last to show signs of an unhealthy lifestyle, and the reverse is true when you remove toxins from the body. But in less than ten to twelve days of removing and detoxing the body of toxins you can expect to see clearer, smoother skin. Skin conditions may also disappear. You may notice your skin itches or gets patchy before clearing up, but this is part of the process. You are on the right track, and will soon experience the benefits of younger-looking skin.

Better Breath – Once the body and colon are free of toxic, smelly buildup, you should start noticing fresher breath. It's been theorized that one contributor to bad breath is a backed-up colon. Again, be aware that your breath may get worse before it get better; this is normal, as toxins are being released from your body.

Brain Improvement – Your gut plays a big role in brain health. Often you will experience less forgetfulness, and be in a better mood. All these are a direct result of a healthy body, healthy brain. Often processed foods contain neurotoxins that affect brain chemistry that causes mood swings, forgetfulness and depression.

Healthier Hair – When your hair is able to get the nutrients it needs through the healthy absorption of vital nutrients, your hair will shine, feel softer, and look healthier. Another benefit you may see is that nails and hair grow faster.

Reverse Aging – Being toxic accelerates the signs of aging and damages skin cells. A poor diet, toxic overload, unbalanced gut, inactivity, and stress are leading causes of premature aging. By eliminating these factors, your body will start to regenerate and heal from an unhealthy lifestyle. The body was designed to regenerate, replace, and rebuild itself. However, all this is impaired by a toxic lifestyle. I like using this example: You can put poor quality gas in your car, but over time, toxic buildup in the form of carbon deposit will collect and clog vital functions and affect the performance of the vehicle, which will break down and stop working.

2. Juice or Blend Anti-Aging Superfoods

There's no denying that juicing or drinking a fruit or vegetable smoothie is a great way to get a large dose of micronutrients into your body. Making anti-aging juices is not difficult. However, in order to look and feel young without going through too much trouble, it is better if beginners stick to easy ingredients and mix and match to taste with in-season, anti-aging superfoods and herbs.

Before you start, understand that these anti-aging superfoods and juice blends are not a magic quick fix to turn back time and make you appear younger in an instant. They do, however, contain powerful the right amount of anti-aging properties that combined with toxic elimination will restore your health, revitalize your mood and energy and reduce the signs of premature aging and wrinkles.

It's recommended that you detox the body before embarking on our *Juice Your Way Back* challenge. Once you have eliminated your daily bombardment of toxins, I recommend a minimum of one to two juices or anti-aging smoothies per day.

3. Eat Organic

Once you're past the detox stage and have started your one to two juices per day, I recommend eating only organic fruits, vegetables, meats, eggs, etc. I know how difficult it is to source, buy, and eat organic at home and on the road. But you need to make it your top priority to eat and juice organic as often as possible and prepare your day to always be thinking, *is this food I'm eating or product I'm using toxic?* The goal is to give your body a break so that it can cleanse and restore old worn out cells with healthy resilient ones. Remember any non-organic, processed food or beverage is toxic. Use this as your motivation to keep yourself toxin-free, and make it your mission to be obsessed with seeking out non-chemical laced foods and products.

Conventional non-organic farming uses chemicals, genetically modified organisms (GMOs) and synthetic products and practices to grow produce faster and at larger volumes, without testing for safety, and often at the expense of consumers' health. When you buy conventional commercially-grown fruits and vegetables, you are buying produce that been sprayed with some of the deadliest, lethal bug killers pesticides and herbicides known to mankind. And all meats are full of toxic, acidic chemicals from what they eat, to what is injected, and the stress they are put though as their growing in small cages before they are brutally slaughtered. Use this as your motivation to keep yourself toxin-free, and make it your mission to be obsessed with seeking out whole food organic grocery stores and restaurants.

4. Stay Hydrated

Your organs cannot function properly if you are dehydrated. Water is one of the most important sources of energy for your body. It helps cells complete important enzymatic activities, which contribute to good sleep, restoration of bodily systems, and the production of ample energy to get you through your day. Water is essential for the proper circulation of nutrients in the body. Water serves as the body's transportation system, and when we are dehydrated things, just can't get around as well.

Here are some of the benefits of keeping well hydrated throughout the day.

Reduce High Blood Pressure – When the body is fully hydrated, the blood is approximately 92% water. This helps to keep the blood moving freely through the veins and arteries, helping to prevent high blood pressure along with other cardiovascular ailments.

Reduce Allergies – When the body is dehydrated, it creates more histamines—organic nitrous compounds which help to regulate our immune response. If we have too many histamines circulating, we will feel congested and have difficulty breathing, along with other allergic reactions caused by the body's response to foreign bodies. Did you know that being well-hydrated can prevent cancer? Yes, that's right—various research says staying hydrated can reduce your risk of colon cancer by 45%[5], bladder cancer by 50%[6], and possibly reduce breast cancer risk as well.

Reduce Acne – Regular and plentiful water consumption can improve the color and texture of your skin by keeping it building new cells properly. Drinking water also helps the skin regulate the body's temperature through sweating. Dermatitis, psoriasis, and premature aging of the skin—proper hydration can reduce most skin problems.

Lower Cholesterol – When the body does not get enough water, it will start to produce more cholesterol so that cells can still function properly. Drinking plenty of water helps cholesterol levels stay in check—along with a proper diet, of course.

Eliminate Digestive Disorders – Water can help eliminate and reduce the incidence of ulcers, bloating, gas, gastritis, acid reflux, and IBS. You also will experience less frequent constipation, since water helps waste move more quickly through the intestinal tract. A well-hydrated body purges toxins and metabolic wastes much more easily. Our digestive system needs water to function properly. Waste is flushed out in the form of urine and sweat. If we don't drink water, we don't flush out waste, and it collects in our body and causes a myriad of problems. Combined with fiber, water can cure constipation.

Flush Out Unwanted Bacteria from the Bladder and Kidneys – People who are well-hydrated experience less frequent bladder or kidney infections, since water helps to flush out any unwanted microbes that try to accumulate in liver and kidneys. These organs are especially sensitive to disease without proper hydration since they are responsible for eliminating stored toxins and bodily waste.

Speed Up Joint and Cartilage Repair – Drinking water can reduce pain in your joints by keeping the cartilage soft and hydrated. This is actually how glucosamine helps reduce joint pain, by aiding in cartilage's absorption of water. Most of the padding in our cartilage is made up of water, so if we don't drink enough water, our bones and joints will feel stiff. Joint repair after workouts or injuries is also improved by proper hydration.

Help with Weight Loss – Sometimes we think we are hungry, but actually we are thirsty. Our body just starts turning on all the alarms when we ignore it. For those of you trying to drop some pounds, staying hydrated can serve as an appetite suppressant and help with weight loss. When our cells are depleted of water, they cannot create energy we need to function, and so they send a signal to the brain to "get more goods." This means you will eat more, and likely carry some extra unwanted pounds. To avoid this, simply stay hydrated and your cells will stay happy and not send 'fat signals' to the brain. Further, and more obviously, replacing other drinks with water will help naturally keep the weight off. Some water with lemon each morning can be especially beneficial.

Help with Mood – Research says dehydration can affect your mood and make you grumpy and confused.[3] Think clearer and be happier by drinking more water. Proper hydration contributes to increased athletic performance as well. Water composes 75% of our muscle tissue![4] Dehydration can lead to weakness, fatigue, dizziness, and electrolyte imbalance. Sometimes headaches can be caused by dehydration, so drinking water can prevent or alleviate that head pain.

Slow the Aging Process – Last but certainly not least, proper hydration slows the aging process and keeps skin healthy and supple. Skin being one of the largest organs in the body, all organs require proper hydration to function properly. If your dehydrated for long periods of time, every cell, organ, and system in the body has to work harder, which means you will age faster. Drinking enough water literally keeps you younger looking, increases energy and vitality–for life.

Tips: Try drinking water with a little lemon after a workout instead of sports drinks that are full of refined sugar, dyes, and chemicals. Instead of drinking soda, drink water. Try adding some lemon, orange or cucumber wedges or even letting a pitcher of water infused with herbs like mint, basil, or sage. Keep in the refrigerator overnight. The result is delicious and nutritious. Bottled water is deceiving. It is less regulated than tap water and costs 2,000 times more. If you're on-the-go, grab a bottle, but otherwise, opt for purified, filtered water.

Avoid Tap Water – Just like eating organic foods, you must also drink purified and/or filtered water and avoid tap water when ever possible. Why do you think that is? Like with non-organic foods, tap water is processed and treated with toxic chemicals that can scar your arteries, and cause heart disease and a whole host of other diseases, when coupled with all the other toxins your body is exposed to on a daily basis. It is best to avoid drinking tap water altogether, to be safe and to avoid additional toxins your body must process out. Alternative solutions may include bottled water, filtered tap water, shower filters, reverse osmosis filters, etc.

I know what you're thinking—I'm a hypochondriacal freak, right? Do your own research and search the Internet yourself. According to a Health Wyze Article, "The Dangers of Tap Water," the water supply in most American cities contains chlorine, fluoride, and varying amounts of dissolved minerals, including calcium, magnesium, sodium, chlorides, sulfates, and bicarbonates. It is also common to find traces of iron, manganese, copper, aluminum, nitrates, insecticides, and herbicides.

Prescription medications have also been found in the tap water in millions of American homes. According to the Associated Press, there is a vast array of pharmaceuticals including antibiotics, anti-convulsants, mood stabilizers, and sex hormones in the municipal water supplies. Think about the millions of people who flush their meds down the toilet. The U.S. government does not require filtering and or any testing for drugs in the water supplies, nor does it set safety limits for drug contamination. It will be decades before we know the long-term effects of ingesting random cocktails of partially digested prescription drugs. Sadly, our grandchildren will know.

It is recommended to drink a minimum of six to eight glasses of filtered or bottled water every day. In addition to our toxic bodies, we are a nation of dehydrated, but functioning, toxic zombies. The average person is under-hydrated. Our bodies are made up of 75% water, and blood is as much as 91% water. You need to drink water. It's instrumental not only in hydration and for flushing and nourishing the body but also in keeping our body's pH balanced.

How to tell if you're hydrated? One of the first things you should do is take a look at the color of your urine. This can tell a lot about how hydrated you are. The perfect color of your urine, if you are well-hydrated, is faint yellow. The darker the yellow, the less hydrated you are. If you don't drink enough water, then your urine becomes over-concentrated with toxic waste, which is why it's a darker yellow. Urine may have a variety of colors. It usually ranges from a deep amber or honey color to a light straw color, with many golden variations in between.

Below is a description of color and condition of hydration and your health.

No Color/Transparent – You're drinking a lot of water. You may want to cut back.

Pale Straw Color – You're normal. Healthy and well-hydrated.

Transparent Yellow – You're normal. Healthy and well-hydrated.

Dark Yellow – Normal. But drink some water soon.

Amber or Honey – Your body isn't getting enough water. Drink some water a.s.a.p.

Syrup or Brown Ale – Possible liver disease/sever dehydration. Drink water. See a doctor if it persists.

Orange – Severe dehydration possible liver or bile duct problem. Possible food dye. See doctor a.s.a.p.

Pink to Reddish – Most likely you have juiced or eaten lots of beets or blueberries recently. If not, you may have blood in your urine from kidney disease, tumor, UTI, prostate, or something else. See your doctor right away.

When the body is not property hydrated, toxins build up, and the body becomes more acidic and susceptible to disease, and the skin sags, wrinkles and discolors. If you don't drink water—maybe a week. Most of us should prioritize the consumption of water far more than we currently do.

Drink Water Upon Waking

From 4:00 a.m. to noon the next day, your system is eliminating toxins in your body. When you wake up, your body is naturally dehydrated, no matter how much water you drank the previous day. Drinking up to two glasses of water upon waking will provide your cells with much needed, life-giving water. You will feel more refreshed, have more energy throughout the morning, and overall be healthier and happier. It will also boost the detoxification process. As you sleep, the body is hard at work clearing itself of toxins, replenishing energy, and balancing hormones.

Give your body a boost by drinking filtered warm water with a squeeze of lemon juice. Lemons contains an antioxidant called dlimonene, which takes compounds present in the liver that are toxic to cells and converts them to non-harmful or less harmful versions. These toxins can range from caffeine to ibuprofen. Aside from the detoxing effect of lemon water and other antioxidant benefits, warm water and lemon juice help fight wrinkles and blemishes while repairing damage from free radicals.

If you don't have lemons, try adding 2 teaspoons of organic apple cider vinegar to a glass of water. This miracle elixir has been known to aid in all types of health benefits, from losing weight, banishing bad breath, protecting your heart, keeping blood sugar levels in check, aiding in digestion and, most importantly, helping to restore alkalinity in the body, which can boost metabolism, strengthen immunity, and slow the aging process to give you clearer, wrinkle-free skin. Visit our website at www.juiceyourwayback.com to learn more about apple cider vinegar.

Before you drink your first glass of water each morning, make sure to wash out your mouth by swishing water around in your mouth and spitting it out, and/or brush your teeth with an all-natural toothpaste. The reason you should wash out your mouth before drinking your first glass of water is that, after sleeping, your mouth builds up bacteria as you sleep. Not cleaning, rinsing, or washing your mouth out before you drink upon waking causes all that bacteria to wash into your stomach which has been known to cause several health issues.

5. *Stop Consuming Sugar*

The United States Department of Agriculture (USDA) reports that the average American consumes anywhere between **150 to 170 pounds** of refined sugars in a year! You may be thinking, "I do not consume that much sugar." Let's break it down. Eating 150-170 pounds of sugar in one year is also equivalent to consuming 1/4 to 1/2 pounds of sugar *each day*. That is 30-60 teaspoons of sugar in a 24-hour period. It only takes four 12-ounce cans of sodas to equal 1/4 pound of sugar!

Americans consume refined sugars in numerous forms—there

are the obvious sugary culprits such as cake, candy, cookies, dough-nuts, and ice cream. However, sugar is hidden in virtually everything we consume daily. Sweeteners such as high fructose corn syrup can be found in barbecue sauces, breads, muffins, canned fruits, canned vegetables, cookies, crackers, frozen dinners, hot dogs, ketchup, marinades, salad dressing, peanut butter, pickles, and soups.

Almost anything processed contains sugar. When food manu-facturers researched what Americans wanted (i.e. low carbs, no fat, no gluten, etc.), they removed these and put in more sugar. Sugar is a legal drug ten times more addictive then cocaine. Don't believe me? Try going cold turkey and see for yourself the symptoms of withdrawal. It is not only a drug—it is a poison, too. It depletes us of our life forces, proteins, minerals and vitamins. We have all heard about the dangers of consuming too much sugar; it can lead to organ malfunction and hormone disruption, resulting in aller-gies, arthritis, behavioral problems, degenerative organ disease, depression, diabetes, immune disruption, migraines, mental illness, obesity, and tooth decay.

How does eating sugar relate to being ill? Excess sugar con-sumption depresses your body's immunity. Studies have shown that consuming 75 to 100 grams of simple sugars (about 20 teaspoons of sugar—the amount found in two-and-a-half average 12 ounce cans of soda) can suppress the body's immune responses considerably.

These sugars are known to create a 40 to 50% percent drop in the ability of white blood cells to kill bacteria and germs within the body. The immune-suppressing effect of sugar starts less than thirty minutes after ingestion and may last for five hours. By consuming 50 to 170 pounds of simple sugars each year, a person may have up to 80,000 hours of immune suppression!

With the average American consuming 50 to 170 pounds of sugar on average annually, I am not surprised to read that worldwide obesity rate has more than doubled since 1980 and that more than 45% of adults across America are categorized as obese.

Note: By going on a detox cleanse and ridding the body of parasites and sugar, you will experience symptoms of withdrawal and side effects, similar to drug or alcohol withdrawal. Below is a list of possible withdrawal symptoms that you may experience when you cut sugar from your diet. It's advisable to replace man-made sugars with natural sugars such as organic fruits to help wean yourself off this drug. When juicing or blending the ratio should 80 percent veggies and 10 to 20% fruits, which should give you the amount necessary to lessen the withdrawals. Not everyone will go through all of the symptoms listed below—withdrawal varies in severity and intensity depending on the person, their level of consumption, size, and weight.

Anger: If you quit cold turkey, your mood may dip, and you may notice that you are more angry and irritable than usual. The anger should not last more than a couple weeks, but may be difficult to cope with if it was unexpected.

Anxiety: Various individuals have reported feeling anxiety when they drop sugar from their diets. It is known that sugar can have an influence on dopamine levels and activity, which could be the culprit for these feelings. Certain individuals are more sensitive than others to experiencing anxiety during the elimination process.

Appetite: Eating sugar can lead some people to experience increased cravings for carbohydrates. Additionally, when you stop consuming sugar, you may notice that your appetite has some degree of fluctuation. Initially you may eat more or less than usual, but it should balance out.

Cravings: When you stop eating sugar, you're going to crave it. These cravings may be intense, and difficult to overcome. If you stay the course, you will eventually reach a point where these crav-ings subside. It may help to remove sugar substances from your house and/or keep them out of sight so that you don't fall victim to the cravings.

Depression: People can experience a crash in mood when they stop eating sugar. This dip in mood is typically not very extreme, but can feel like a low-grade depression. Eventually your mood should lift again and stabilize.

Dizziness: In more extreme cases of withdrawal, individuals have reported feeling dizzy when they stop consuming sugar. Most people will not feel "dizzy" when they stop including sugar in their diets, but more sensitive people may.

Fatigue: Sugar can provide some people with short-term boosts in energy. When a person quits including sugar in their diet, it is possible to experience some general fatigue and lethargy during the first couple weeks of withdrawal. Over the long term, a person should notice that normal energy levels return.

Flu-like Symptoms: In some cases, people actually experience a severe reaction to cutting sugar from their diet that results in very low-grade, flu-like symptoms. If you have this severe a reaction, it should subside within a few days. Most people will not experi-ence this particular symptom when they cut sugar, but everyone is affected differently.

Headaches: Initially some people experience headaches when they remove sugar from their diet. These headaches can be a result of tension and/or the changes you are going through by detoxifying your body from sugar.

Insomnia: Dropping sugar from your diet may temporarily result in changes in sleep patterns and arousal. You may notice that you are unable to fall asleep at a proper time because you feel anxious or your arousal level has changed; this will eventually go away. Consider taking melatonin or using some sort of relaxation exercise before bed if it's a big problem.

Irritability: Early on, you may become snappy as a result of not having the sugar that you crave. Sugar can influence dopamine, a neurotransmitter responsible for pleasure in the brain. When we are no longer getting the same stimulation, we may become irritable.

Mood swings: It is fairly common to experience minor mood swings when you initially cut sugar from your diet. The mood swings may consist of some minor depression, anxiety, and/or other negative feelings. Eventually your moods will stabilize on their own, but it may take a short while for your brain to adjust.

Shakes: In some cases, people can actually shake when they drastically cut their sugar consumption. These shakes are usually a result of cold turkey withdrawal, but are typically not too severe; they will eventually subside. This is actually a fairly common symptom among people who stop consuming sugar that were previously consuming high amounts.

Weight changes: Most people notice that they lose weight when they drop sugar consumption. Weight loss is generally due to the fact that people stop consuming sugar-filled foods and beverages. There is no exact science suggesting that sugar withdrawal takes a specific amount of time. The duration for which you experience withdrawal symptoms will largely depend on you as a person. Some people are able to quickly adjust to functioning without sugar, while others may have a difficult time resisting cravings and the feelings that they get when they have something sugary. Based on various experiences, most people do notice that they go through some sort of a withdrawal period when they drop sugar from their diet. However, the length of this withdrawal period is subject to variation. Some people felt considerably better and were virtually withdrawal symptom free within a few days, while it took others a full month to feel completely detoxified.

When you stop consuming sugar, your dopamine levels may temporarily drop – leading to various psychological symptoms. To help address this problem, it is recommended you consume lean protein, fruits, and nuts for additional nutrients. It is also recommended to avoid sugar-replacement products, as these substances act similarly on the brain and can also have eerily similar discontinuation symptoms. Additionally, if you are a big soda drinker and/or like energy drinks, you could also be experiencing caffeine withdrawals—this is something to consider.

The good news is that incorporating our fruit, vegetable and herbal blends into your daily diet will help you get though withdrawal and will shorten the time of withdrawal. Once you have cleared the symptoms you'll start to notice a body that is more efficient and may notice the following: weight loss, your hair, skin and nails begin to radiate and glow with health and vigor. Your energy levels may increase while depression, stress, anxiety and fatigue significantly reduce. Food cravings will also decrease.

6. Stop Eating Processed Foods

If it comes in a package, it's processed. Look at the ingredients. If it says things you don't recognize or can't pronounce, don't eat it. Only choose organic whole foods and meats. There are over fifteen thousand chemicals food manufacturers are not required put on labels. Do not trust any fancy packaging or marketing phrases like fat free, carb free, sugar free, low sodium, light, healthy, all natural etc. Remember these are all marketing

tricks to get you to buy. For example one of the largest soup companies in the world just got busted for advertising "low sodium"
plastered in bold on the front of the can. When in fact the sodium
content was the same if not more than their regular option. So
why wouldn't they take the sodium out, you would think they
could save money and give consumers what they want. The real
reason is taste. Someone going from a high-sodium diet to half
the salt would never purchase that product again because it taste
terrible and they know that. So they deceive the public in hopes
they will sell more product based on the latest fads.

Another deceptive trick they use is put in super small amounts
of a healthy ingredient then display it prominently in bold big
letters i.e. Omega-3s, Antioxidants, Whole Grains, Natural, or
Vitamin Enriched, to name a few. This is purely a marketing
trick. The amounts of these nutrients are often negligible and
do nothing to make up for the harmful effects of the other toxic
ingredients. The unfortunate sad truth is major corporations are
forced to keep shareholders happy, so they can receive their hefty
bonuses. Food fraud, mislabeling and deception is a widespread
epidemic, and rarely policed or regulated. To remain profitable
these companies often substitute their products with man-made
inexpensive excitoxins chemicals, flavor enhancers and artificial
sweeteners to increase their profits and get you addicted.

Instead buy organic, all natural, handmade, locally grown
meats and produce. I know this sound crazy, but if you are ded-
icated to looking and feeling your best and youngest, you will
learn there are a ton of foods choices that are at your local grocery store that are 100% natural or organic—all of them delicious,
and chemical and toxin free. Of course, it's best to just avoid processed foods altogether, and eat **real foods** instead, that way you
don't have to worry about labels and ingredients lists. Real food

doesn't even need an ingredients list…real food *is* the ingredient.

Processed meats are bad for you too—they might even cause cancer. New research shows a direct link between eating processed meats multiple times a week and cancer and heart disease, according to a recent study published in BMC Medicine. The European Prospective Investigation into Cancer and Nutrition (EPIC) study looked at health effects on half a million men and women in ten different countries. The researchers found a link between processed meat consumption and increased chance of early death, especially from cardiovascular disease and cancer.

So what exactly are processed meats? Any type of meat that has been processed or manipulated, other than being cut or ground from its natural state. Non-organic meats in general are loaded with hormones, chemicals and antibiotics as it is, but food processors add flavoring, chemical preservatives, and dyes, and mix them with less desirable parts of an animal to increase its taste and volume yield. Processed meats include canned meats, cured meats, any type of lunch meat, sausage, hot dog, bacon, or anything with a casing or in a sausage form, or anything smoked or cured.

According to the study, poultry like chicken and or duck will not increase your odds of cancer or cardiovascular disease. They suggest buying sliced chicken instead of pre-packaged, processed meats. The key link is the chemicals used in the processing of these products. Look for unprocessed or organic meats whenever possible. Look for meats that offer hormone- or nitrate-free products. For example, buy a turkey breast and roast it at home to save on the preservatives.

For protein options other than processed meats, try foods like tuna, eggs, fish, lentils, beans, nut butters, tofu or organic plant base protein powders (hemp, whey or soy) to get your recommend daily allowance of protein. Which according to The DRI (Dietary

Reference Intake) is 0.8 grams of protein per kilogram of body weight, or 0.36 grams per pound. This amounts to **56 grams per day** for the average sedentary man and **46 grams per day** for the average sedentary woman.

7. Stop Smoking

Smoking is the leading cause of aging prematurely and introduces highly addictive chemicals and toxins that cause cancer. Smoking affects your ability to get a full night's rest. According to a Johns Hopkins study, smokers are four times more likely than nonsmokers to report feeling less rested after a night's sleep. Smoking also causes bags to appear under your eyes. If you smoke, you will be more likely to get Psoriasis, an autoimmune related skin condition. Smoking also stains your teeth, fingers, and nails.

Smoking is the leading cause of premature aging and wrinkling. It also causes the skin cells to dry out and die, discoloring the skin through vitamin depletion. As if wrinkly skin, nails, and teeth weren't enough to motivate you to quit, toxic chemicals in smoke can damage the DNA in hair follicles, resulting in premature hair loss. Smoking causes scars and wounds to take longer to heal, because of restricted blood flow. Smoking puts you at risk of dental problems, including tooth loss. Smokers are also more susceptible to infection, skin cancer, bad breath, and stretch marks, because smoking damages the fibers and connective tissue in your skin. Cigarette smoking can also increase your risk of cataracts. Smoking causes a 22% increased risk of cataract extraction, according to one study. It's never too late to quit.

8. Take Probiotics

If your gut bacteria is filled with unfavorable microorganisms, you are putting your body at risk for disease and premature aging due to the body's inability to fight off toxins and age-related disease.

Over 85% of humans suffer from unhealthy unbalance of good bacteria in their gut. This imbalance causes an overgrowth in our gut of bad fungus called *candida*, a yeast-like, parasitic fungus that can sometimes be called thrush. It's a parasitic worm that hijacks your body and can break down the walls of the intestine and enter into your bloodstream, releasing toxins into your body and causing one of the most common issues today: leaky gut. If you've ever taken perception medication or antibiotic, these fast-growing unfavorable parasites overrun your gut. For example, did you know that an inch of uncooked salmon contains over 10,000 parasite larva, and that over 1/3 of our stools is not even from you, but from the waste of parasites that are living in your digestive system?

Before you start a diet program or juicing nutrition program, you must get your gut under control. One of the chemicals parasites release sends signals to the brain, causing you to crave the foods they live on, like sugars, sodas, junk foods, and high-carbohydrate sweets. If you don't push back and build up the good bacteria in your intestinal system, you are wasting time getting fit, reversing the signs of premature aging, and restoring your health. Besides making passable stools, good gut bacteria (called probiotics) also synthesize vitamins B-7 (biotin), B-12, and K. The deficiency of these essential vitamins contributes to diabetes, obesity, hair loss, gray hair, eczema, premature aging, seborrhea, anemia, internal bleeding, ulcers, strokes, cancers, degenerative disorders such as Parkinson's and Alzheimer's disease, and common gastrointestinal, respiratory, and autoimmune disorders.

If you are currently taking or have taken antibiotics, eaten any Genetically Modified Corn (GMO), which is sprayed with antibiotics, corn syrup, or any processed corn by-product, drink tap water your bacteria balance (good vs. bad bacterial balance) is compromised. GMO corn is sprayed and treated with antibiotics.

In addition, non-organic meats are routinely given antibiotics. When you consume or drink these processed food products that have been treated with antibiotics, it destroys your digestive good bacteria, causing an imbalance in your digestive health.

Other factors that disrupt the balance of your intestinal bacteria include:

- Inorganic antibiotic residues in meat and dairy products
- Chlorinated and fluorinated water
- Continual stress
- Diets high in sugar and simple carbohydrates (like fast food and junk food)
- Estrogen replacement
- Exposure to radiation (CAT Scans, excessive medical X-Rays)
- Oral contraceptives
- Parasites
- Poor digestion/constipation
- Toxic chemical intake

Still think your gut isn't out of balance or that you don't have parasites?

Do you suffer from one or any of these conditions—constipation, bloating, diarrhea, irritable bowel disease, difficulty in losing weight, acid reflux, peptic ulcers, toe fungus, white coated tongue, bad breath, gum disease, itchy skin, or rashes? Do you often get colds, the flu, and infections, have chronic fatigue, anemia, infertility, acne, eczema, hair loss, premature graying, premature wrinkles, pre-diabetes, diabetes, neurological damage, intestinal disorders, oral sores, asthma, seborrhea, poor sleep patterns, nightmares, or extreme menstrual or menopausal symptoms?

Probiotics are the good bacteria in your digestive system that help stimulate the natural digestive juices and enzymes that keep our digestive organs functioning efficiently. It is virtually impossible to kill all the parasites in your gut. Your goal, however, is 80% good bacteria and 20% bad bacteria to get your digestive system to function normally. People that have incorporated a candida cleanse or taken probiotics have seen their health restored. They have dropped weight easily and had their energy restored. Again, you must include these helpful bacteria in your system before you start any cleanse or juicing program. Otherwise, juicing will not be as effective. Probiotics help digest food, protect us from pathogens, (dangerous micro-organisms), help detox harmful chemicals and toxins, and produce vitamins and other vital nutrients and balance out your immune system. 70% to 80% of the cells that make up the immune system come from your gut.

In my experience and research, taking probiotics is extremely important to your health and appearance. However, the fastest and best way to populate your gut with good bacteria is by taking a dual-capsulation acid resistant probiotic. If you eat any consumable probiotic products (i.e. yogurt or kefir), your stomach acid destroys most if not all of the good bacteria before it even enters the gut. Taking a probiotic supplement lets it bypass stomach acid and has a minimum of 15 billion CFUs, or cultivated forming units or individual good bacteria. Bypassing the acid and delivering lots of good bacteria daily will have enormous benefits for your health and appearance.

For a list of probiotic supplements that use this type of delivery system and CFUs, visit my website at www.juiceyourwayback.com/supplements/cbtl.

9. Eliminate All Artificial Sweeteners and MSG

Avoid all artificial sweeteners, such as Nutrasweet or Splenda, and MSG, or monosodium glutamate. Even if it's not on the label, it's most likely added. The FDA does not require manufacturers to label these foods as containing MSG unless the "added ingredient" is 99% pure MSG.

Other names for MSG are hydrolyzed vegetable protein, textured vegetable protein, yeast extract, glutamic acid, glutamate, calcium glutamate yeast food, soy protein, whey protein, calcium caseinate, sodium caseinate, or anything with the name glutamate. In summary, MSG is a flavor enhancer found in processed food and is most likely under "aliases" so it's impossible to know what you're eating.

All artificial sweeteners and chemical flavor enhancers are classified as excitotoxins, which are a class of chemicals that over-stimulate neuron receptors in the brain, causing them to become exhausted and/or depleted. These are all chemically manufactured sweeteners and flavor enhancers, which have been shown to cause many diseases, including but not limited to Alzheimer's, Lou Gehrig's Disease, depression, MS, headaches, asthma, epilepsy, heart irregularities, ADD, and hyperactivity disorders—to name a few. If you're one of the tens of millions of Americans who needs a sugar fix, try organic coconut palm sugar, organic raw blue agave, or organic vanilla sugar, all of which are available at local health food stores.

10. Don't Drink Diet or Zero-Calorie Sodas

All diet sodas and drinks contain artificial chemicals. Diet drinks and carbonated drinks block calcium absorption in the body, which can affect insulin resistance, cause glucose intolerance, increase cardiovascular disease, inflammation, risk of Type 2 diabetes, and (the big shocker) cause rapid weight gain.

Diet drinks contain artificial sweeteners called NutraSweet or aspartame (methyl alcohol which, when digested, is converted into formaldehyde). These chemical sweeteners can make calorie-free drinks up to 200 to 600 times sweeter than sugar.

But your body doesn't know the difference, and alerts certain transmitters in the body, such as a sense of fullness or satisfaction. If your body thinks it's getting too much sweetness, it will start the conversion to fat process, because it's tricked into thinking you have an overabundance of calories. It gets worse as you get older.

As you age, your metabolism slows down and will accelerate your waistline's expansion much more than if you did not drink diet drinks. These are just a few reasons sodas are the most consumed beverage worldwide. They trick the body and cause you to be addicted to the powerful sugar rush, even though it's chemically produced and contains caffeine.

11. Throw your Microwave Away

While I understand that microwaves are a quick, easy way to heat or reheat food, they are killing all the cells in your food by using over 2.4 gigahertz (Ghz) of frequencies. Your cell phone only uses about 1850-1990 Mhz, and there is plenty of research which states that excessive cell phone use may lead to brain cancer. No organic cell can withstand the radiation effects of a microwave. A study in the Science of Food and Agriculture looked at the effects of microwaving food. Broccoli, for example, lost over 97% of its antioxidants vs. steamed broccoli, which only lost 11%.

The chances are that anything that is microwavable and comes in a box is most likely processed and chemically-laced, toxic, and void of live nutrients. By microwaving your food, you are killing anything that was remotely healthy and/or alive, and adding radiation poisoning to boot.

Another study from a Swiss food scientist, Hans Hertel, found that microwaving food led to a negative impact on physiology and the heart. After studying the effects of microwaved foods, Hertel concluded that microwaving food led to food degeneration. These degenerative changes in nutrients caused changes in the blood that caused health problem such as elevated cholesterol levels, plummeting white blood cell levels, decreased red blood cell levels, production of radiolytic compounds, and decreased hemoglobin levels, which might indicate anemia.

There is no reason to use a microwave, especially when comparing the benefits to the risks. If you want a quick meal in the same time it takes to nuke a TV dinner, juicing is the ultimate fast food. By freezing your organic juice in ice cube trays, you can have healthy, life-giving, age-rejuvenating meals in less than sixty seconds.

12. Stop Using Toxic Products

The idea behind restoring your youthful glow and appearance is to eliminate as many toxins in your body as possible. This will give your liver and kidneys the chance to remove what you cannot control. Below are just a few toxic products that should be substituted with alternative health natural ones. You should be aware of the products you are using on yourself and your children, and practice looking for all-natural, organic, chemical-free alternatives.

Toothpaste: The FDA requires poison warning labels on toothpaste because toothpaste contains a greater concentration of fluoride than tap water. Fluoride is a by-product of industrial waste. Manufacturing companies thought that they would sell this to utility companies, since it was so costly to dispose of and added it to water to dispose of the costly toxin. Since natural fluoride can slow down tooth decay, dentists and toothpaste manufacturers became a part of the plot. Fluoride is still recommended by dentist as a preventative measure for tooth decay.

Sodium fluoride, found in commercial toothpaste, causes demineralization by removing the calcium from teeth, which in the long term discolors them and makes them brittle. Other ingredients used in toothpaste are just as toxic. Saccharin, for example was banned in the 70s because it proved to cause severe health problems in rats. However, that problem was excused because of the taste.

Toothpaste today is especially dangerous, with all the flavored toothpastes marketed to children, such as bubble-gum, fruit, and candy-like flavors. Children are often not aware of the dangers, and don't think twice about swallowing this paste, thus becoming susceptible to illness and fluoride poisoning over time. Risks from ingesting fluoride toothpaste or being absorbed through micro-abrasion from aggressive brushing include permanent tooth discoloration, stomach ailments, acute toxicity, skin rashes and impairment in your glucose metabolism. Fluoride toothpastes sold today contains between 1,100 and 1,450 parts per million (ppm) fluoride (the equivalent of over 1 milligram of fluoride per each gram of paste). It's not surprising that a number of studies found that many children ingest a significant amount of fluoride each day from toothpaste alone, according to the Journal of Public Health Dentistry.

Look for fluoride-free toothpaste. It's not worth the risk to your health and your children's. For a list of safe, non-fluoride based, all-natural toothpaste alternatives, go to my website www. juiceyourwayback.com.

Deodorants: Studies in recent years have linked aluminum-based antiperspirants to a significant increase to breast cancer. According to the authors of these studies, most breast cancers develop in the upper outer part of the breast—the area closest to the armpits, which is where antiperspirants are applied. Blood and lymph vessels serving the arm travel through the armpit. There are more than twenty lymph nodes (small lumps of tissue that are part of the body's lymphatic system, which helps fight infection) in the armpit. These lymph nodes normally cannot be felt through the skin.

The studies suggest that chemicals in antiperspirants, including aluminum, are absorbed into the skin through the armpit and make their way into the lymph nodes when the skin is cut during shaving. These studies claim that those chemicals may then interact with DNA and lead to cancerous changes in cells, or interfere with the action of the female hormone estrogen, which is known to influence the growth of breast cancer cells. The goal of looking and feeling younger is to reduce as many toxins in any one given day. Choose organic deodorants.

For a list of safe, non-aluminum based organic deodorants, go to my website www.juiceyourwayback.com.

Cleaning Wipes: It seems counter-intuitive to use toxic chemicals to wipe down your oven, floors, counters, and toilets to get them "clean." Corrosive or caustic cleaners, such as the lye and acids found in drain cleaners, oven cleaners, and acid-based toilet bowl cleaners, are the most dangerous cleaning products in the world because they burn skin, eyes, and internal tissue easily. There are a ton of non-toxic cleaners you can buy or make on your own using basic household ingredients.

Oil-based Paints and Finishes: There are 300 toxic chemicals and 150 carcinogens potentially present in oil-based paint, according to a John Hopkins University study. To be sure you and your children are not exposed to toxic paint and fumes look for water-based options instead—ideally those that are low- or no-VOC. Volatile organic compounds are organic chemicals that have a high vapor pressure at ordinary room temperature. Their high vapor pressure results from a low boiling point, which causes large numbers of molecules to evaporate or sublimate from the liquid or solid form of the compound and enter the surrounding air. Other options for wood finishes include all-natural finishes like milk, paint, and vegetable or wax-based wood finishes.

Bottled Water: Americans buy half a billion bottles of water every week, according to the documentary film *The Story of Bottled Water*. Most people buy bottled water thinking they're avoiding any contaminants that may be present in their tap water. For the most part, that's not true. Bottled water can be just as, or even more, contaminated than tap water. In fact, some bottled water is simply attractively packaged tap water. Non-BPA plastic bottles can leech chemicals into the water. Also, from manufacture to disposal, bottled water creates an enormous amount of pollution, making our water even less drinkable. Do yourself and the world a favor and invest in a reusable stainless steel water bottle, water filters, or use only BPA-free bottles and plastic to reduce toxin overload for you and your children.

Cosmetics: Your skin covers your body and acts as a physical barrier to many of the pollutants in the atmosphere. When you use makeup on your skin such as cosmetics, lotions, and shampoos, the chemical ingredients in these products are absorbed directly into your body. You may ask yourself where the ingredients in the products go. Modern research at the Herb Research Foundation found that the skin absorbs up to 60% of the chemicals in products that it comes into contact with. The chemicals go directly into the bloodstream. Today, hormone therapy treatments and smoking cessation medications are often prescribed as patches applied directly to the skin. The medication passes through the skin and enters the bloodstream.

For pregnant women, the risk also extends to the developing fetus. If the chemicals found in cosmetics readily enter the bloodstream when applied to the skin, then they will also reach the developing baby. Researchers at the Brunel University in England are looking closely at a family of preservatives called parabens. Their research has recently linked parabens to the possibility that male babies will have lower sperm counts. These preservatives are derived from petroleum and help to maintain the freshness and integrity of the product. Currently, many manufacturers add parabens to cosmetics to allow a minimum of a three-year shelf life. Therefore, the parabens kill any bacteria that could potentially enter the product. If these chemical ingredients can kill the bacterial cells, what are they doing to your skin cells? In most cases, there is no conclusive answer to this question. However, research strongly suggests that the synthetic ingredients may have a significant impact on our bodies.

In many cases, the long-term effects of many of the chemical additives in our cosmetics are not known. However, other chemical additives are known carcinogens. These types of chemicals can cause cancer in humans. Such chemicals include some artificial colors in cosmetics. The effects of chemicals and other synthetic ingredients in cosmetics may lead to mild allergic reactions causing rashes and minor skin irritation to more significant problems such as lesions on the skin.

Luckily, there are alternatives to cosmetics filled with synthetically produced ingredients. Increasingly, cosmetic manufacturers are answering the public's demand for alternatives to the chemically loaded beauty and grooming supplies. For a list of all natural cosmetics companies leading the way in producing high-quality, organically manufactured cosmetics. Visit my website at www.juice-yourwayback.com As a consumer, you have the ability to decrease the number of preservatives and toxic chemical additives your skin comes into contact with and therefore enter your body that adversely affect your health. To avoid using the synthetically derived fragrances, look for products containing essential oils. These are pure oils derived from flowers and other plants in nature.

All you have to do is make the simple choice of purchasing cosmetic products with all-natural, organic ingredients. Whether you continue using cosmetics that contain petroleum-based ingredients or not is a personal choice. What is the most important is to get the facts, and to know that you have a choice when it comes to buying organic or synthetic cosmetic products.

Lead Lipstick: This one shocked me. Did you know that lipstick often contains lead? Lead is a known neurotoxin that has no safe level of exposure—and is found in lipsticks. A study by the U.S. Food and Drug Administration discovered lead in 400 lipsticks tested, two times more than were found in a previous FDA study. There is no safe level of lead exposure. Pregnant women and children are at risk especially, since lead can interfere with normal brain development.

Triclosan: A toxic antibacterial agent often found in soaps, toothpastes, mouthwashes, deodorants, and even clothing. Studies have shown that triclosan may harm the immune system, which may make you more likely to develop allergies and weakness. Yet another example of a toxic chemical still in use despite overwhelming proof if its dangers. The FDA warns consumers to read labels for triclosan and recommends using plain soap to clean up. Instead of using antibacterial hand sanitizers made with triclosan, choose an alternative made with at least 60% alcohol.

Fragrance products: Fragrances found in everyday products like air fresheners, dryer sheets, and perfumes may trigger asthma because of the toxic chemicals used to produce the product. Some of the chemicals mimic estrogen, which may increase the risk of breast cancer. For example, diethyl phthalate (DEP) can accumulate in human fat tissue if not eliminated. Phthalates are suspected carcinogens and hormone disrupters that are increasingly being linked to reproductive disorders. To be safe, choose fragrance-free products or use those scented with natural fragrances like essential oils.

Parabens: Unquestionably, the most commonly used in the cosmetics industry. A preservative made from toxic, petroleum-based end product, Parabens are in just about any cream you rub, put on your lips or apply to your skin. Parabens are used to prevent mold, fungus, and parasites from growing. Parabens are also often found in breast cancer tumors! All signs point to skin care products being the cause. Because of this, there is a growing concern that excessive use of parabens may increase breast cancer in women and testicular cancer in men. Although there haven't been any conclusive studies proving this, it should be enough to make you concerned. In fact, it's why there are so many "paraben-free" items popping up in the supermarket and pharmacies around the country.

Parabens can appear in different forms, so here's what you want to look out for:

- benzylparaben
- butyiparaben
- propylparaben
- methylparaben
- ethylparaben
- isobutylparaben

Phitalates: These are found in just about everything—even you. A recent study done by the US CDC found a trace of it in every single person they analyzed. This is problematic because phthalates—which are used in cosmetics and also in many plastic objects—have been found to act as a hormone disrupter linked to reproductive defects, insulin resistance, and developmental problems in children. As mentioned, most chemicals don't need to be listed on products, and phthalates aren't listed on the label of your favorite products either, so you have to do a bit of research to determine their presence. Here's a tip. They're often found in anything that lists "fragrance" as an ingredient. Look for alternative products that use essential oils instead.

Benzoly Peroxide: Benzoyl peroxide is used in acne-treatment medications, which has been proven to be a cancer-causing agent and has received FDA warnings for potentially life-threatening side-effects. Moreover, benzoyl peroxide takes a vicious approach of attacking skin to reduce problem areas, rather than nourishing it with nutrients, hydration, and all-natural ingredients.

Perhaps most startling is the long-term deleterious effects of benzoyl peroxide on the body. Studies have shown that benzoyl peroxide generates free radicals in skin. Free radicals cause oxidative stress on cells and damage DNA, both of which may result in cancer. Because of this genetic code degradation, benzoyl peroxide has been linked to cancer, especially skin cancer, and has been deemed a "tumor promoter."

Moreover, even when benzoyl peroxide may succeed in reducing acne or other skin conditions, it may impede overall skin care goals. Oxidative stress damages cells and slows the healing process. It can result in a longer recovery from acne than other natural skin care methods like apple cider vinegar, coconut oil, tea tree oil, lemon juice, garlic or aloe. But worst of all, it can cause premature aging and or skin cancer. The more benzoyl peroxide used, the more damage it can do to skin on a long-term basis.

Resorcinol: One of the most common ingredients in bleaches and dyes. Resorcinol is a known skin irritant that has been shown to disrupt healthy thyroid function in animals. It's also a common cause of allergic reactions to hair dye. This chemical is absorbed into your scalp.

Hydroquinone: Is used as a skin lightener that reduces dark blemishes. Hydroquinone reduces the melanin in your skin to get rid of those unsightly marks, but in doing so, it damages your skin in many ways. First of all, it's permanently alters your pigment while also weakening the elastin and collagen in your problem area – the very things that are key to keeping your skin firm, elastic and youthful! Some people get unsightly blotches after using this toxic chemical, and far more get contact dermatitis or have allergic reactions after regular use.

Petroleum: Health effects from exposure to petroleum products vary depending on the concentration of the substance and the length of time that one is exposed. Breathing petroleum vapors can cause nervous system effects (such as headache, nausea, and dizziness) and respiratory irritation. Very high exposure can cause comas and even death. Liquid petroleum products, which come in contact with the skin, can cause irritation, and some of it can be absorbed through the skin. Chronic exposure to petroleum products may affect the nervous system, blood, and kidneys. Gasoline contains small amounts of benzene, a known human carcinogen. Animals exposed to high levels of some petroleum products have developed liver and kidney tumors. Whether specific petroleum products can cause cancer in humans is not known, but there is evidence that occupationally exposed people in the petroleum refining industry have an increased risk of skin cancer and leukemia.[6]

It hides behind many names that you should familiarize yourself with. They are:

- Petrolatum
- Xylene
- Toluene
- Mineral oil
- Liquid paraffin

Methylisothiazolinone: Also known as MIT, methylisothiazolinone is an increasingly common antibacterial preservative, found in everything from baby shampoo to moisturizer. Studies have shown that it contains neurotoxic properties. In studies with rats, a mere ten minutes of exposure to MIT was enough to cause brain cell damage. Further studies concluded that low concentrations of MIT during neural development increased the risk of seizures and visual abnormalities.

Even though the amount found in most products is small, and meant to be rinsed off, our bodies are so toxic that unless the body removes it, which is virtually impossible since we are generally already in toxic overload, these chemicals will build up in your fat cells and cause mutation, leading to diseases and serious side effects.

Oxybenzone: Functions as a photo stabilizer and sunscreen ingredient that absorbs UVB ray. Found in most sunscreen lotions and cosmetics as a preservative, protecting the product from deteriorating under the sun. According to the Environmental Working Group, there are several suspected dangers associated with Oxybenzone. Despite its abilities to protect against the sun, it has been shown to penetrate the skin and cause photosensitivity. As a photocarcinogen, it increases the production of harmful free radicals and an ability to attack DNA cells; for this reason, it is believed to be a contributing factor in the recent rise of Melanoma cases with sunscreen users. Some studies have shown it to behave similarly to the hormone estrogen, suggesting that it may cause breast cancer. It has also been linked to contact eczema and allergies.

In addition, there exist many concerns regarding the human body's absorption of Oxybenzone. In one study, individuals applied a sunscreen with 4% Oxybenzone and submitted urine samples 5 days after topical application. All the subjects' urine secretions were found to contain Oxybenzone, suggesting the body's ability to store the substance. In 2008, the US Centers for Disease Control & Prevention conducted a similar experiment on a national scale, and found the chemical compound to be present in 96.8% of the human urine samples surveyed. As a result, it is recommended that parents keep their small children from using products containing the ingredient. This is based on the assertion that children under the age of two have not fully developed the enzymes that are required to break down derivatives of Oxybenzone.

Artificial Dyes: Whether you're donning a hot pink lipstick, a classic rouge, or a rebellious black nail polish, if your favorite cosmetics are conventional, chances are they are just as dangerous as they are fabulous. Many of the products you have are likely made with synthetic colors made from coal tar. Though pretty, these harsh artificial colors have been shown in to be carcinogenic and are likely to cause skin sensitivity and irritation due to the heavy metals they deposit on your skin.

13. Stop Using Non-Stick or Teflon-Based Cookware

Did you know that when using non-stick cookware at certain temperatures, leeching of the chemical coating occurs and it becomes fumes? This is because the non-stick cookware is made using a carcinogenic chemical called perfluorooctanoic acid also know as (PFOA), which are released as toxic fumes every time you cook at high temperatures. 90% of Americans have PFOA in their blood. One of the reasons for such a high percentage is that the chemical remains in your body for quite some time, often for years, before your body can process out these chemicals. There is no doubt that non-stick cookware is dangerous to your health. This may come as a shock to you, but know this: the scientific evidence is absolute. There are a lot of alternatives for safe cookware besides non-stick, PFOA-treated cookware. Alternatives include aluminum-based, stainless, coated, or non-coated cookware. These will not release toxic fumes.

14. Avoid Eating Farm-Raised Fish

Industrial fish farming, or aquaculture, is one of the fastest growing food productions in the world. About half of world's seafood now comes from aquaculture. For the first time in our planet's history, farmed fish processing has surpassed beef production. And fish farmers, just like so many agricultural farmers, add chemicals, hormones, and additives that preserve the meat and produce larger quantities without a concern for the side effects to your health. They often use the cheapest, genetically modified foods to feed farm-raised fish, and inject the fish full of antibiotics, hormones, and chemicals. For example, farmed raised salmon are fed pellets, chicken fat or skin, soy meal, etc. Because they've been raised on this processed food diet, their flesh turns gray. Chemical dye is then used to color the salmon pink, so it looks like wild caught salmon according to an article in The Atlantic, March 2015. Wild salmon gets its pink skin color from krill in the ocean, not processed pellets.

Like birds and mammals, fish feel pain and stress, and are subject to the same inhumane practices as land animals, like living in very tightly confined environments. Then they are killed by evisceration, starvation, or asphyxiation. These days, even salmon raised on farms is being packaged and sold as wild. With the dyes and clever marketing, you may never be able to tell the difference. And these food manufacturers are often not required by law to disclose or include all the ingredients listing on the packaging. As discussed, food mislabeling and fraud runs rampant amongst food manufacturers looking to deceive and profit from our lack education of what's going on behind closed doors. One way to tell if your salmon is farm-raised or wild caught is under the ingredient list, look for any dyes or colorings that are used. Again remember they are not required by law to list all the additives and chemicals used, which may not include the dye used to make the salmon look pink. Consumers think the deeper the pink color, the fresher the product, and food manufacturers and processors know this and simply add more dyes to sell more product.

15. Stop Eating Canned Foods

Whenever you apply heat to food, its vitamin and enzyme potencies are diminished. This also applies to boiling, processing, and preserving foods. Canned foods are largely empty calories with little to no nutritional value, and are loaded with sodium. They are attractive to consumers because of their convenience. A French scientist initially came up with the idea in the nineteenth century, as a stopgap to stave off death by starvation on the battlefield.

Here are some reasons canned food must be eliminated from your diet:

1.   The major concern is that it is often treated with BPA poisonous chemicals. Most canned foods today have a plastic lining

inside the can that is treated with BPA-treated plastic. BPA kills rats in laboratories even in smaller portions 1000 times less than what an average American consumes per meal.

2.   Imported canned food is even worse than American canned foods, for two reasons. Firstly, they have to make the canned food much cheaper and less nutritious because of the additional shipping cost. Only 2% of imported canned food is inspected by FDA, the Homeland Security Agency, or any other organization (e.g. EPA for environmental monitoring). You have no idea what's in the cans or cheap chemicals used to process the product when you consume canned foods.

3.   Even worse is that aluminum-canned foods are often cooked in the cans and sealed—supposedly to preserve freshness. This is a huge concern, because whenever you heat something, the chemical composition changes and is often absorbed by the product. Aluminum accumulation in the body can, over time, cause memory loss, Alzheimer's and cancer.

4.   Canned foods are treated with preservatives. Although there is no proof that chemicals used in foods and products cause death and disease in small doses, your body is overwhelmed with toxins and chemicals every day, and cannot process them all out of your body. Unless you make drastic changes to prevent them from entering your body, they will be stored and over time you will age prematurely and will become sick.

In summary, avoid canned foods at all cost. In the event you do use a canned food product, always look for organic products and/or products in glass jars.

16. Stop Taking Vitamins

Have you ever taken vitamins on an empty stomach? Taking multivitamins on an empty stomach can sometimes cause nausea and an upset stomach. Copper and iron can often cause such ill effects in the amount present in multivitamins. Similarly, acidic vitamins like vitamin C and vitamin B-3 can also cause nausea and an upset stomach. High concentrations of acidic vitamins can be toxic to your stomach; there's no denying that prolonged deficiency of certain vitamins can lead to illness and disease. The real question, though, is whether vitamin supplements are necessary for *healthy* individuals.

If you eat and/or juice a diet full of fruits and vegetables, there's a good chance you've already reached your suggested daily intake. And even if you eat a less-than-stellar diet, many types of processed foods are fortified with vitamins and minerals.

The best way to correct any vitamin, mineral, or enzyme deficiency is by eating more plant-based foods, and by juicing. The second-best way, if your diet doesn't give you the daily recommended allowances, is to consider taking an all-natural, organic, whole-food-based multi-vitamins or all natural supplements which are made of plant-based fruits and vegetables, not synthetically made in a laboratory.

Studies have found that a daily multivitamin won't help boost the average American's health, the experts behind the research are urging people to abandon use of vitamins. The studies found that popping a daily multivitamin didn't ward off heart problems or memory loss, and wasn't tied to a longer life span. The studies, published in the Dec. 17 issue of the journal *Annals of Internal Medicine*, found that multivitamin and mineral supplements did not work any better than placebo pills.

A growing body of evidence suggests that multivitamins offer little or nothing in the way of health benefits, and some studies suggest that high doses of certain vitamins may cause harm. "We believe that it's clear that vitamins are not working," said Dr.

Eliseo Guallar, a professor of epidemiology at the Johns Hopkins Bloomberg School of Public Health. It's not clear that taking supplements to fill gaps in a less-than-perfect diet really translates into any kind of health boost. "It would be great if all dietary problems could be solved with a pill," he said. "Unfortunately, that's not the case."

In addition, by taking over the counter vitamins today, do you really know what you're getting? If they are made by a "for profit" company, keep in mind their main purpose is profit, not purity of product. There have been many companies busted for either substituting ingredients, or putting in tiny amounts of what the label shows. Recent cases were against WMT, GNC, Target, and Walgreen's, which all removed the misleading supplements from their shelf.

"The probability of a meaningful effect is so small that it's not worth doing study after study and spending research dollars on these questions," Guallar said.

17. Stop Eating Shellfish and Sushi

Shellfish is delicious, but hardly a health food. In fact, shellfish and sushi are among the most toxic, parasitic foods on the planet. Shellfish feed on carcasses, which are often disease-ridden and contain a host of parasites and man-made chemicals. The problem with these bottom feeders is their digestive systems are not designed to filter out the toxins and parasites, meaning anything they eat that is toxic or contains parasites stays in their bodies and is never eliminated, and then is consumed by humans.

Mercury and many other contaminates are often found in shellfish as well. Mercury is one of the most hazardous of the heavy metals and may cause serious health problems. This is probably why more people are allergic to shellfish than any other food, more people get sick from eating shellfish than any other food on the planet, and more people die from eating shellfish and sushi than any other food.

Sushi contains harmful chemicals, parasites, and eggs, and are packed full of calories, fat, and salt. Sushi contains a cocktail of chemicals, heavy metals, small worms, and pesticides, which can potentially lower intelligence, reduce fertility, and even lead to cancer. "If you eat a meal of salmon sushi more than twice a year, you will increase your risk of cancer," says Professor David Carpenter, an environmental health scientist at the University at Albany, New York. "People think they're improving their health by eating sushi but they are, in fact, poisoning themselves," says Professor Carpenter. Raw fish often contains herring worms, nematodes, or roundworms, and can result in severe abdominal pain, nausea and vomiting within hours of consuming raw fish or sushi. Often these symptoms are misdiagnosed as appendicitis or other stomach problems and diseases. If the worms don't get coughed up or expelled through vomiting, they can burrow into the walls of your intestines and cause localized immune responses.

Shellfish to avoid are lobsters, crawfish, crayfish, langoustines, prawns, crabs, mussels, whelks, winkles, clams, cockles, scallops, and oysters.

Raw fish and sushi to avoid that are high in mercury are yellowfin and bluefin tuna, horse mackerel, any yellowtail, bonito, swordfish, blue marlin, mackerel, young sea bass, and albacore tuna.

18. Eat Food Cooked at a Low Temperature, or Raw

When you consume foods/drinks processed or cooked at high temperatures, your body is exposed to a process called mutagens or advanced glycation end products (AGEs). This is the chemical process that happens when you consume processed foods and/ or foods cooked at high temperatures. The high heat mutates the structure of the food cellular properties and damages the cellular integrity of your DNA once consumed, causing the cells in your body to be susceptible to cancer and accelerating the aging process of your entire body. As AGEs build up in the body, they damage the cellular engines—the mitochondria. The loss of cellular energy gives rise to a dizzying array of age-related complaints such as loss of memory, hearing, vision, and stamina. Even more troubling are new findings that show AGEs accumulate in the arterial plaque of people with heart disease as well as in the brains of those with Alzheimer's and Parkinson's disease. They also have a hand in cataract formation.

The measurements for glycation products, or AGEs, are measured in Kilounits (KU/serving). Below are the worst culprits, foods that should be avoided at all cost. For a complete list of food products that cause the biggest risk to your health when consuming them or cooking go to my website www.juiceyourwayback.com.

Chicken skin, back, or thigh, roasted then BBQ – 16,668 KU

Bacon, fried five minutes no added oil – 11,905 KU

Broiled beef hot dogs – 10,143 KU

Pan-fried beef – 9,052 KU

Big Mac (MacDonald's) – 7,801 KU

Grilled beef – 6,674 KU

Pork-link sausage – 5,349 KU

* The above AGEs KU per serving are from an article in the Aug. 2015 issue of *Life Extension* magazine. Live longer by changing how you cook.

Foods cooked at high temperatures with low moisture content are the greatest risk to your body. Cooking the foods using lower temperatures, poaching, steaming, stewing, or boiling will lower the glycation process of the proteins in the food.

19. Stop Tempting Yourself

One of the hardest things to do is have control over your food choices, both at home and on the road. With parasites highjacking our hormones and craving impulses and advertisers bombarding us morning, noon, and night, it's best not to temp yourself and buy junk food or processed food treats and have them in your home, car or office.

Stop kidding yourself that you will only eat one or two treats and then put them away. Success all starts at the grocery store, with what you put in your basket. Soon these cravings will pass, and you will start getting sick when you eat these toxic treats. Once this happens you will be truly on your way. Instead of ice cream, freeze bananas or other fruits, and snack on healthy treats instead.

20. Stop Showering in Tap Water

Last but not least are the toxic dangers of showering without water filters. Tap water is filled with toxic chemicals. The problem is, the skin is the largest organ and absorbs anything running over or rubbed into it. The real concern is when water becomes heated and steams, chemicals in the unfiltered water become airborne and enter your lungs, which is a direct path to your blood supply. It's like being in a toxic gas chamber. "Chlorine is used almost universally in the treatment of public used water because of its toxic effects on harmful bacteria and other waterborne, disease carrying organisms. But there is a growing body of scientific evidence that shows that chlorine in drinking water may actually pose greater long-term dangers than those for which it was used to eliminate the toxic bacteria and viruses.

Researchers have now proven that it is unhealthy to shower or bathe in chlorinated and/or polluted, unfiltered water. It is a real danger, say the experts. These effects of chlorine may result in either ingestion or absorption through the skin. Scientific studies have linked chlorine and chlorination by-products to cancer of the bladder, liver, stomach, rectum, and colon, as well as heart disease. Since chlorine is required by public health regulations to be present in all public drinking water supplies, it is up to the individual to remove it at the point-of-use in the home."

As mentioned, when you shower or bathe, chemicals in the water vaporize, releasing poisonous gases from volatile organic compounds. This literally transforms the bathroom into a mini gas chamber, filling it with toxic gases such as chlorine— a chemical used as a poisonous gas during World War I.

Chlorine attacks organic matter. It has been proven to be a major cause of cancer and has been linked to many diseases such as heart disease and birth defects. Because it chemically bonds with body proteins, it commonly causes brittle and dry hair, red, itchy, burning eyes, and many skin problems, such as dry skin, red itchy skin, and different types of dermatitis.

Think about this way: Diluted chlorine is toxic enough to kill all living organisms in the water. How could it not affect humans in some harmful way? Furthermore, like other volatile organic chemicals, it becomes even more dangerous once it is vaporized and absorbed into the lungs and enters your blood system.

According to the Ralph Nader report, one inhales and absorbs **100 times** the amount of chemicals from the water by showering or bathing than one would by drinking the same amount of water.

Even the EPA, after devoting so much effort to the secondary smoke issue, is now studying the carcinogenic (cancer-causing) effects of taking unfiltered showers and baths. Once its findings are made public, nearly everyone will want a shower and bath filter.

However, since overwhelming evidence about the harmful effects of chemicals in shower and bath water already exists, why endanger your health by waiting for a "Johnny-come-lately" EPA to confirm the obvious?

For a list of BPA free shower filters go to my website www.juiceyourwayback.com.

Be a Role Model and Inspire Others

One thing I have discovered is the infectiousness of learning, leading by example, and inspiring others during and after their *Juice Your Way Back* lifestyle. Educating and inspiring others is by far the most rewarding aspect of my work. You too will have the power to pay it forward with the knowledge you'll gain from this book. As you learn and share your experiences and your journey with others, they will most likely want to join you in your quest to look and feel better. Join me in educating and inspiring others, and your life will be enriched. You will also be motivated to continue learning, living, and feeling your best.

"To know even one life has breathed easier because you have lived. This is to have succeeded."
—Ralph Waldo Emerson

CHAPTER 6

FOUNTAIN OF YOUTH SUPERFOODS

ANTIOXIDANTS

Antioxidants play an important role in our overall health and appearance. They are natural compounds found in some foods that help neutralize free radicals in our bodies. Free radicals are substances that occur naturally in our bodies but attack the fats, protein, and DNA in our cells, which can accelerate the aging process and onset of diseases.

Aging and disease are a result of accumulated toxins and chemicals in your body. These chemicals cause cellular damage, brought on by free radicals or molecules that have become unstable after losing one of their orbiting electrons. In an attempt to restore balance, free radicals will steal electrons from other molecules, causing damage through a process called oxidation.

Antioxidants protect the body against excessive oxidation by neutralizing free radicals, and, accordingly, play a major role in the prevention of these conditions associated with their retractions. Free radicals are reduced through normal metabolism in the body but increase with exposure to modified animal flesh, processed foods, alcohol, cigarettes, and radiation, as well as chemical pollutants found in water, air, and food. Out of all the things we are exposed to, the one we have the most control over is providing our bodies high antioxidant-rich foods in our daily diets. Juicing is an ideal method of consuming high levels of these essential antioxidants.

Through experimentation and extensive research, below is a list of the most effective and antioxidant-rich fruits, vegetables, and herbs to achieve the fastest anti-aging cellular regeneration results possible. It is paramount to bring these to your attention because the foundation of reversing damaged skin and restoring health are primarily found in these powerful "superfoods," and should be incorporated into your daily diet.

Bioflavonoids are a group of water-soluble elements that help maintain the strength and proper function of the capillaries. Along with vitamin C, bioflavonoids help manufacture collagens, which are the building blocks of our entire body and are the most abundant protein in the human body. Bioflavonoids also protect cells against attack from viruses and bacteria.

Foods – grapes, rose hips, green teas, oranges, lemons, cherries, parsley, cabbage, apricots, peppers, papayas, tomatoes, broccoli, raspberries, and blackberries.

Glutathione (pronounced "gloota-thigh-own") is the most important molecule you need to stay healthy and prevent aging, cancer, heart disease, dementia, and more. It is necessary to treat everything from Autism to Alzheimer's. I call it the mother of all antioxidants. The good news is that your body produces its own glutathione. The bad news is that toxins from poor diet, medication, stress, trauma, aging, infection, pollution and radiation all deplete your glutathione causing the liver to become overloaded and damaged, and thus unable to do its job, leaving you susceptible to cell disintegration from oxidative stress and free radicals.

Foods – spinach, broccoli, kale, collards, asparagus, garlic, avocados, cabbage, cauliflower, watercress and bananas.

Resveratrol (pronounced "res-ver-a-trol") a polyphenol compound found in certain plants and in red wine that has antioxidant properties. Resveratrol is a very powerful antioxidant that provides greater protection against DNA damage than even Vitamin C or E. Resveratrol and its antioxidant properties also help immensely in repairing the damage caused by oxidizing agents. Thus a healthy level of antioxidants, like vitamin C, vitamin E and selenium, are essential to prevent chronic inflammatory damage, arrest pre-cancerous changes, and slow the so-called aging changes.

Foods – skins of red and white grapes, peanuts, pistachios, mulberries, blueberries, cranberries, and even found in cocoa and dark chocolate.

Selenium (pronounced "se-le-ni-um") is an antioxidant. Its primary function is to protect cells from destruction. Selenium plays a vital role in the enzyme system and is necessary for the manufacture of prostaglandins, which controls blood pressure and blood clotting. Selenium also protects eyes against cataracts, contributes to protein production, and protects the artery walls from plaque buildup.

Foods – Brazilian nuts, mushrooms, asparagus, broccoli, onions, and tomatoes.

Vitamin A is fat-soluble, and essential for healthy bones and teeth, sperm production and formation, epithelial growth in skin cells and tissue, and vision health. It's one of the most powerful vitamins for the maintenance of the body's immune responses, which helps the body fight off infection. It is essential for maintaining healthy skin and protects the mucous membranes of the lungs, throat, mouth, and nose. Vitamin A also helps the body secrete the gastric juices necessary for protein digestion and protects the lining of the digestive tract, kidneys, and bladder.

Foods – carrots, beets, greens, spinach, sweet potatoes, winter squash, lettuce, dried apricots, cantaloupe, bell peppers, fish, liver, and tropical fruits.

Vitamin C promotes cell regeneration and is one of the most powerful immune system and detoxification agents. Diets high in vitamin C protect the body against cardiovascular disease and various forms of cancer, maintains mental health, and may even prolong life. The presence of vitamin C is necessary to build collagen. Vitamin C combats the toxins introduced to our body, and is a natural laxative.

Foods – papayas, bell peppers, dark leafy greens, broccoli, peas, strawberries, pineapples, kiwis, oranges, lemons, sprouts, sweet potatoes, and kale.

Vitamin E maintains cellular strength and promotes skin and muscle health. It protects our fatty acids from destruction. This vitamin is the major nutrient used by our bodies to protect against environmental stress. It helps dilute the harmful effects of consuming lead, excessive minerals such as sodium, or the otherwise unbalanced mineral content of most drinking water.

Foods – almonds, raw seeds, Swiss chard, spinach, turnip greens, kale, hazelnuts, organic eggs, pine nuts, avocado, broccoli, parsley, papaya, and olives.

Zinc is an essential mineral required to maintain a sense of smell, keep a healthy immune system, building proteins, triggering enzymes, and creating DNA. Zinc also helps cells communicate by functioning as a neurotransmitter. A deficiency in zinc can lead to stunted growth, diarrhea, impotence, hair loss, eye and skin lesions, impaired appetite, and depressed immunity. Zinc helps combat viruses and bacteria and is essential in the formation of stomach acid.

Foods – sunflower seed, pumpkin seeds, sesame seeds, cocoa powder, wheat germ, spinach, cashews, and mushrooms.

ENZYMES

Enzymes are biological molecules (typically proteins) that speed up the rate of chemical reactions within cells. They are vital for life and serve a wide range of important functions in the body, such as aiding in digestion and metabolism.

Some enzymes help break large molecules into smaller pieces that are more easily absorbed by the body. Other enzymes help bind two molecules together to produce a new molecule. Enzymes are highly selective catalysts, meaning that each enzyme only speeds up a specific reaction.

But because the modern human diets consist of mostly cooked, enzyme-depleted foods, the body's ability to synthesize the quantity and kind of enzymes needed to keep us healthy and our immune systems functioning is compromised. The body naturally produces enzymes, but when you get sick, stressed, injured, depressed, or older, the body produces less and less enzymes, causing you to get sicker or develop serious illnesses and diseases. This is why you must be diligent in incorporating enzyme-rich foods in your diet as you age.

Enzymes are found in large quantities in fruits and vegetables. It is important to note that heat destroys enzymes. If you have to cook fruits or vegetables, cook them below 115 degrees Fahrenheit and just long enough to slightly soften the vegetable or fruit. If you don't have access to fresh organic fruits or vegetables, frozen produce is the next best option. However, freezing fruits temporarily inactivates enzymes, so try to use organic fruits and vegetables, whenever possible. Also, sprouts contain high amounts of enzymes and minerals, and you can easily grow them indoors.

Below is a list of some powerful enzyme-rich superfoods

Papaya

Papaya fruit is a rich source of proteolytic enzymes such as papain, which can aid the digestive process. Papain is effective at breaking down meat and other proteins. It works by splitting the peptide bonds of complex proteins, breaking them down to their individual amino acids so they can be ready to use in the growth and repair of the body. Since papaya is rich in natural sugars, it's a good idea to eat it on its own, preferably fifteen to thirty minutes before a meal.

Pineapple

Bromelain is a complex mixture of substances that can be extracted from the stem and core fruit of the pineapple. Among dozens of components known to exist in this crude extract, the best-studied components are protein-digesting enzymes called cysteine proteinases. These enzymes are not limited to just digestive benefits, but as research has shown, they also help with excessive inflammation, excessive coagulation of the blood, and certain types of tumor growth. Since pineapple is also rich in natural sugars, it is a good idea to eat it on its own, preferably fifteen to thirty minutes before a meal.

Bee pollen

Bee pollen is often considered one of nature's most complete foods. It contains nearly all the nutrients required by humans and has abroad spectrum of beneficial enzymes including amylase, catalase, cozymase, cytochrome, dehydrogenase, diaphorase, diastase, pectase, and phosphatase. Bee pollen can be eaten on its own or put in trail mixes, oatmeal, superfood snacks, and smoothies. Bee pollen can cause allergic reactions, so be mindful of that when trying it for the first time.

Fermented vegetables

The fermentation process used to make sauerkraut and kimchi was developed centuries ago as a means of preserving vegetables for consumption through the winter months. The Roman army was said to have traveled with barrels of sauerkraut, using it to prevent intestinal infections among the troops during long excursions.

Fermented vegetables are an excellent dietary source of many nutrients, including live enzymes (provided they have not been pasteurized in any way). These live enzymes are accompanied by beneficial probiotics, which makes an exceptional combination for an effective digestive process.

Fermented vegetables can be eaten on their own, but they also go great with any meal as a side. In fact, if you want to improve the digestion of any meal, you should strongly consider a side of fermented vegetables.

Other enzyme-rich foods to consider include melons, mango, kiwi, grapes, avocado, raw honey, kefir, wheat grass juice, and coconut water.

HERBS

As mentioned, organic fresh juices of plants from herbs, fruits, or vegetables will have the greatest potential to reverse disorders and aging. By using organic plants, results will be even better. In most cases, herbs have not been hybridized or genetically altered the way that so many of our processed foods have today. Fresh plants are nature's enzyme storehouses. Herbs and vegetable juices are one of the best ways to restore an individual back to health, as well as increase our enzyme reserves. The higher our enzyme reserves, the greater our chances of living a long and healthy life. One of the most powerful herbs, known for its anti-aging properties as well as its ability to increase vitality, stamina, vigor, and to reverse premature greying of the hair is called He Shou Wu.

He Shou Wu – also known as Fo-Ti root, this herb has been used in traditional Chinese medicine for over three thousand years and is known throughout Far East as the "Elixir of Life". Considered one of the most potent anti-aging, rejuvenation and longevity herbs.

He Shou Wu has other amazing benefits—it is an effective anti-anxiety, mood enhancer, and stress reduction herb. As you know stress, is the number one killer, and the number one cause of disease and accelerated aging. He Shou Wu has a long history of use as a medication prescribed for the treatment of depression.

Other benefits of this herb include an abundant supply of iron and zinc, which are essential trace minerals and play a vital role in the growth and development of our immune response. They also aid in neurological function and reproduction. Zinc is a very effective vitamin for sexual and reproductive functions. He Shou Wu root is also very useful to older individuals who may suffer from common joint health issues.

Suggested Use: Mix 1 tablespoon with juice, probiotic Kefir, or yogurt, or add to your favorite smoothie, or mix into a tea.

Before using He Shou Wu:

Do not take this herb is you are pregnant or nursing. Tell your doctor or pharmacist if you have any medical conditions, or if you have or used to have liver disease.

Bilberry – Bilberries are small blue berries rich in antioxidants. Research suggests that these berries are an incredible defense against early signs of aging, including wrinkles and scars. They also reportedly promote healthy vision and eyes; this is especially beneficial for those concerned about macular degeneration and cataracts. With their potent antioxidant activity, the bilberry herb protects body tissues, particularly blood vessels, from oxidizing agents circulating in the blood. In fact, bilberries contain the highest antioxidant level, bite for bite, of any berry! In the same way that pipes rust as a result of an attack by chemicals, various chemicals in our environment—pollutants, smoke, and chemicals in food—can bind to and oxidize blood vessels. Antioxidants allow these harmful oxidizing agents to bind to them instead of to body cells, preventing the agents from causing permanent damage to the lining of blood vessels.

Before using bilberry:

Some medical conditions may interact with bilberry. Tell your doctor or pharmacist if you have any medical conditions, especially if any of the following apply to you:

- you are pregnant, planning to become pregnant, or are breast-feeding
- you are taking any prescription or nonprescription medicine, herbal preparation, or dietary supplement
- you have allergies to medicines, foods, or other substances
- you have diabetes

Some medicines may interact with bilberry. However, no specific interactions are known at this time.

This may not be a complete list of all interactions that may occur. Ask your health care provider if bilberry may interact with other medicines that you take. Check with your health care provider before you start, stop, or change the dose of any medicine.

Ginseng – The two most common forms of ginseng we see in the west are American ginseng and Asian ginseng. Both are excellent at helping the body physiologically adapt to different needs. This helps fight the effects of stress on the body... and that's just one of the numerous benefits of this herb. Increased stamina and heightened mental and physical performance are also commonly reported.

PROBIOTICS

Below is a list of superfoods that will put this life-giving, age-reversing bacteria back into your gut. Remember to always consume probiotic foods at the beginning of a meal or on a empty stomach for maximum benefits and results. Dairy probiotics and superfood probiotics should be taken during or right after a meal, preferably first thing in the morning or with breakfast.

Organic Yogurt – Only choose unsweetened yogurt, and blend fresh organic fruits in instead. Again, make sure you read the labels carefully and choose only non-GMO products.

Organic Milk – Only choose non-GMO, rBGH-free milk products. Also try to choose unsweetened milk to avoid putting additional sugar into your system. Other milks that may contain probiotic benefits are soy, almond, and coconut milk.

Cultured Cottage Cheese – Not all products and brands include live cultures. Read the label carefully and choose organic if possible and non-GMO.

Kefir – One of the most powerful probiotics on the planet. Kefir is a cultured, creamy product similar to drinkable yogurt, with amazing health benefits. You can make this at home by purchasing kefir starter kits, or buy it pre-made at your local grocery store. Look for kefir products that are free from *all* synthetic hormones and antibiotics, including rBGH and rBST. Look for products that are organic and from grass-fed cows. If you have milk allergies, you can purchase non-dairy water kefir starter kits or kefir grains that you can mix with non-dairy milk products such as, rice milk, soymilk, coconut milk, or almond milk.

Non-Dairy Probiotics

Kombucha Tea – Made from fermented yeasts and bacteria, this yields a carbonated, probiotic-rich drink. Found at your local health food store or occasionally in organic markets.

Miso – Composed of soybeans in combination with barely or rice, miso is a traditional condiment often used in soups and seasoning vegetables, meats, and fish. Found at your local health food store or Chinese market.

Kimchi – Kimchi is a raw vegetable (usually cabbage) fermented in puree of fruit, garlic, ginger, and spices. It's crunchy and very similar to fermented sauerkraut, but spicier. It is Korea's national dish.

Micro Algae – This refers to superfood ocean-based plants such as spirulina, chorellia, and blue-green algae. These plant-based probiotics foods have been shown to increase the amount of probiotics in the digestive tract. They also offer the most amounts of energetic benefits per ounce. Take these types of probiotics in the morning for added energy and probiotic benefits.

Tempeh – A great substitute for meat or tofu, tempeh is a fermented, probiotic-rich grain made from soybeans. A great source of vitamins, this vegetarian meat replacement can be sautéed, substituted for sandwich meat, baked or crumbled on salads. If prepared correctly, tempeh can also be low in salt, which makes it an ideal choice for those on a low-salt diet. Can be found at Trader Joe's, Whole Foods, or other health food stores.

Fermented Sauerkraut – This is loaded with probiotics, vitamin C, and B vitamins. The process of fermenting cabbage actually creates isothiocyanate — a chemical group formed by substituting the oxygen in the isocyanate group with a sulfur thought to inhibit the formation of cancer and tumors.

Water Kefir – Alternatively known as tibicos and Japanese water crystals, water kefir is a probiotic beverage similar to Kombucha and ginger beer. Water kefir grains create a carbonated lacto-fermented beverage from water, fruit juice or coconut water. You can buy these starter kits online or from your local health food store.

Ginger Beer – Ginger beer, much like water kefir, offers a healthy, wholesome alternative to soda. Ginger beer has a naturally fizzy constancy similar to soda and is loved by children.

Dark Chocolate – This might be one of the tastiest items on the list, and it's a surprise to many to find out that dark chocolate is a probiotic food. It also contains a high level of antioxidants. When purchasing dark chocolate, choose from a range of 55% to 85% cacao and, of course, always select organic.

Sour Pickles – Sour pickles are a traditional alternative to vinegar pickles, and are prepared using a simple solution of unrefined sea salt and clean, chlorine-free water.

Probiotic Supplements – Eating or juicing probiotic foods is extremely helpful in providing a balance of good gut bacteria. However, your stomach acid kills a lot of the good bacteria before they make it to the gut. If you're short on time, a time-released or dual encapsulation probiotic is recommended. These have a special coatings or uses unique technology that protects the healthy life-giving bacteria and releases them once they have traveled past the stomach and into your gut.

If you choose to swallow the pill, it is best taken on an empty stomach, about forty-five minutes before breakfast and at night about two hours after your last meal. This allows the capsule time to bypass stomach acid and open or dissolve in the intestinal tract, providing maximum benefits.

For the best probiotic supplement, visit my website at www. juiceyourwayback.com/supplements.

*Probiotics should not interfere with other medicines or natural remedies. It is advised you drink plenty of water while taking a course of probiotics.

CHAPTER 7

ORGANIC VS. TRADITIONAL

O nce found only in health food stores, organic foods and products have recently created a bit of a dilemma in the grocery store aisles. On one hand, you have a traditionally grown apple. On the other, you have one that's organic. Both apples are firm, shiny, and red. Both provide vitamins and fiber, and both are free of fat, sodium, and cholesterol. Which should you choose?

People often say that healthier foods are more expensive, and that such costs strongly limit better diet habits. The healthiest diets cost about $1.50 more per day than the least healthy diets, according to new research from Harvard School of Public Health (HSPH). The finding is based on the most comprehensive examination to date comparing prices of healthy foods and diet patterns vs. less healthy ones. So it's true that an organic diet is a more expensive diet.

It is also true that organic foods are better for you

Of the many benefits of fresh, natural, or organic foods, there are a few things that should be said about fruits and vegetables and their specific benefits. In general, fruits are considered fresh. However, most fruits are picked well before they are ripe, sometimes as long as six weeks. On the other hand fruits targeted for the frozen food isles are allowed to ripen longer. The problem with fruits picked days or weeks ahead of time is they never get a chance to fully achieve their full vitamin and mineral potential. Therefore, by the time you consume them their virtually nutrient void of any meaningful benefit other than a sugar rush. So it's better for your health to include more veggies in your juice or smoothie routine, since most fruits are often lower in vitamin content since they were picked prematurely.

Purchasing fruit picked when ripe is best for maximizing the benefits of the fruit. Find local, organic farms that don't have to pick their fruits so far in advance.

So what does the word "organic" really mean? Organic refers to the way farmers grow and process agricultural products, such as fruits, vegetables, grains, dairy products and meat. Organic farming practices are designed to encourage soil and water conservation and reduce pollution.

Farmers who grow organic produce don't use conventional methods to fertilize and control weeds. Examples of organic farming practices include using natural fertilizers to feed soil and plants, and using crop rotation or mulch to manage weeds.

A number of studies have been completed regarding the effects of antioxidants derived from organic foods on your overall health, and the predominant results have shown that antioxidants tend to have more of an impact when they come from organic foods. This may be due to the fact that foreign chemicals are not negatively interacting with the different vitamins, minerals, and organic compounds that are so essential for the positive impact of fruits and vegetables in the prevention of things like cancer, heart disease, premature aging, vision problems, and cognitive malfunction. Recent research suggests that choosing organic food can lead to increased intake of nutritionally desirable antioxidants and reduced exposure to toxic heavy metals.

One of the major complaints that organic food consumers list when choosing organic over traditionally grown produce is the presence of pesticides and herbicides. In order to keep crops from being attacked by bugs, chemically based pesticides are used. Although they do a good job keeping certain pests away from the crops, they also are composed of powerful chemicals. This is an unnatural mineral compound that is not required by humans, but more than 80% of this material in our bodies comes from eating pesticide-coated foods. Pesticides have been connected to a number of developmental health problems, including autism and ADHD, so organic food makes more sense for small children and older adults. To be fair, many people do choose to go organic to make sure that their children grow up healthy and unaffected by toxins.

In recent decades, one of the biggest projects for farmers and food growers has been genetic modification foods (GMO). Experts say 60 to 70% of processed foods on U.S. grocery store shelves have genetically modified ingredients. Many major crops like corn, soybeans, and tomatoes are grown using genetically engineered seeds. Making tomatoes six times larger might sound like a great option to solve world hunger issues, but there is another side to it. Genetic modification is still in its early stages, so the long-term effects of it on human health aren't well understood. In animal testing, genetically modified food showed a major reduction in immune system strength, an increase in birth mortality, as well as an increase in certain sexual dysfunctions, cancers, and sensitivity to allergens. Although there are some good things about genetically modified food, organic food advocates point to the lack of concrete details about the long-term effects. Organically grown foods do not use pesticides or GMO in the production of crops.

Antibiotic Resistance – People are very sensitive to issues of their health, and they often take precautions to make sure they remain healthy, like getting various vaccines and taking antibiotics as soon as a new strain of bacteria makes them ill. However, non-organic food sources, particularly livestock and feed houses, also use antibiotics to feed their animals. This extra dose of antibiotics from our food and water supply may actually be weakening our immune system by basically overdosing us on antibiotics, thereby reshaping our immune system so many times that it will eventually be unable to defend itself. Organic food growers and dairy farmers do not use antibiotics in their processes.

Overall Health – Since organic food is not prepared using chemical fertilizers, it does not contain any traces of these strong chemicals and might not affect the human body in negative ways. Natural fertilizers, like manure, work perfectly fine, and organic farmers are happy to use this smellier, yet safer, form of fertilizer.

Better Taste – Some people strongly believe that organic food tastes better than non-organic food. The prominent reason for this belief is that it is produced using organic means of production. Furthermore, organic food is often sold locally, resulting in availability of fresh produce in the market, which usually does taste better than produce that has been frozen, shipped, and transported across long distances.

Environmental Safety – As harmful chemicals are not used in organic farming, there is minimal soil, air, and water pollution, thus ensuring a safer and healthier world for future generations.

Animal Welfare – Animal welfare is an important aspect of producing organic milk, organic meat, organic poultry, and organic fish. People feel happy that the animals are not confined to a miserable caged life when they eat organic animal products.

Do "Organic" and "Natural" Mean the Same Thing?

No, "natural" and "organic" are not interchangeable terms. You may see "natural" and other terms such as "all natural," "free-range," or "hormone-free" on food labels. These descriptions must be truthful, but don't confuse them with the term "organic." Only foods that are grown and processed according to USDA organic standards can be labeled organic.

Organic Food: Is it More Nutritious?

Probably not, but the answer isn't clear yet. A recent study examined the past fifty years' worth of scientific articles about the nutrient content of organic and conventional foods. The researchers concluded that organically and conventionally produced foods are not significantly different in their nutrient content. Furthermore, organic food is often sold locally, resulting in availability of fresh produce in the market, which usually does taste better than produce that has been prematurely picked, frozen, shipped, and transported across long distances.

Many factors influence the decision to choose organic food. Some people choose organic food because they prefer the taste. Yet others opt for organic because of concerns such as pesticides, food additives, or environmental concerns.

Food Safety Tips

Whether you go totally organic or opt to mix conventional and organic foods, be sure to keep these tips in mind:

Select a variety of foods from a variety of sources. This will give you a better mix of nutrients and reduce your likelihood of exposure to a single pesticide.

Buy fruits and vegetables in season when possible. To get the freshest produce, ask your grocer what day new produce arrives. Or buy food from your local farmers market.

Read food labels carefully. Just because a product says it's organic or contains organic ingredients doesn't necessarily mean it's a healthier alternative. Some organic products may still be high in sugar, salt, fat, or calories.

Wash and scrub fresh fruits and vegetables thoroughly under

running water. Washing helps remove dirt, bacteria and traces of chemicals from the surface of fruits and vegetables. Not all pesticide residues can be removed by washing, though. You can also peel fruits and vegetables, but peeling can mean losing some fiber and nutrients.

MUST-BUY ORGANIC

The list below contains foods you should buy organic, due to the fact that the pesticides, herbicides, and fungicides used on them are absorbed from the soil, and cannot be washed off.

Fruits and Vegetables

- Apples, grapes, cherries, lemons, limes, oranges, pears, domestic blueberries
- Raspberries, celery, cherry tomatoes, cucumbers, grapes, hot peppers, bell peppers
- Kale, collard greens, all salad greens, peaches, imported nectarines, beets, carrots
- Cucumbers, green beans, potatoes, winter squash
- Potatoes, spinach, strawberries, bell peppers, squash

Nuts, Seeds and Legumes

- Almonds, peanuts, pecans, all soy products, and tofu

DON'T NEED TO BUY ORGANIC

The list below depicts the foods you do not need to buy organic, which either contain small trace amounts of treated chemicals and/or pesticides, or are not as effected by toxins. However, even these foods must be washed thoroughly before eating or juicing.

If you can, always buy local or at farmers markets.

Fruits and Vegetables

- Asparagus, broccoli, Brussels sprouts, cauliflower,

cabbage, garlic

- Avocados, cabbage, cantaloupe, imported blueberries, cantaloupe, onions
- Bananas, grapes, grapefruit, tangerines, mangoes, water-melon
- Sweet Corn, eggplant, grapefruit, kiwi, mangos, mush-rooms, tomatoes
- Onions, papayas, pineapples, frozen sweet peas, sweet potatoes, zucchini

Nuts, Seeds and Legumes

- Beans, cashews, macadamia nuts, sesame seeds

* While it's best to buy organic all the time, go to www.juicey-ourwayback.com to print out a safe grocery list for the next time you go shopping for produce.

CHAPTER 8

KEEPING PRODUCE FRESH

There's nothing worse than loading up on fresh organic produce to find them languishing limply in your crisper drawer days later. To keep produce fresher for longer, follow these tips.

1.   Some fruits and veggies produce a gas called ethylene as they ripen. This gas can prematurely ripen foods that are sensitive to it, so keep ethylene-producing foods away from ethylene-sensitive foods. Avocados, bananas, cantaloupes, kiwis, mangoes, nectarines, pears, plums, and tomatoes, for example, should be stored in a different place than your apples, broccoli, carrots, leafy greens, and watermelon.

2.   Keep potatoes, onions, and tomatoes in a cool, dry place— but not in the fridge. The cold will ruin their flavor.

3.   Store unripe fruits and veggies like pears, peaches, plums, kiwis, mangoes, apricots, avocados, melons, and bananas on the counter. Once they're ripe, move them to the fridge. Banana peels will turn dark brown, but that won't affect the flesh.

4.   Store salad greens and fresh herbs in bags filled with a little air and sealed tightly. Putting a little water in the container and shaking it up, then putting a paper towel on top and lying the produce upside-down revitalizes the spinach and increases the life of the produce. Only add a little bit of water, though; too much will have the opposite effect.

5.   Citrus fruits such as oranges, tangerines, lemons, and limes, will do fine for up to a week in a cool, dark place, away from direct

sunlight, but you can lengthen their lives by storing them in the fridge in a mesh or perforated plastic bag.

6. Wrap celery in aluminum foil and store it in the veggie bin in the fridge.

7. Other types of produce such as carrots, lettuce, and broccoli start to spoil as soon as they're picked, so juice these as soon as possible and fresh to preserve them, or place them in separate plastic baggies in the crisper in your fridge ASAP (make sure they're dry, since moisture speeds up spoiling).

8. Cut the leafy tops of your pineapple off and store your pineapple upside down. This helps redistribute sugars that sink to the bottom during shipping, and also helps it keep longer.

9. Avoid washing berries until right before you're ready to eat them. Wetness encourages mold growth.

10. If you like to wash, dry, and cut your fruits and veggies all at once, store them in covered glass containers lined in paper towels. You'll not only be able to see them—which reminds you to eat them—but you'll also be keeping moisture out.

11. If you normally forget to use up fruits and veggies when you put them in the crisper, store your veggies in plain sight in reusable produce bags that mimic your crisper's function.

12. Buy only what you need. Go to the market more frequently, or if that's not possible, plan out your meals ahead of time so you only buy what you know you'll use.

13. If you notice any rotten produce, compost it immediately before it starts to spoil the rest of the produce.

14. Freeze extra produce to preserve potency. Freezing produce is a great option to stop the aging process. Fruits that are great to freeze include bananas, peaches, strawberries, blackberries, blueberries, etc. Leafy greens are also great to freeze like watercress, kale, spinach, chard, etc. It's best to use frozen produce when blending.

15.　One of the best products to reduce ethylene gas and extend the life of your produce is the Bluapple®. It's designed to provide effective ethylene gas absorption for three months in a typical home refrigerator produce bin or storage container. The active ingredient does not "wear out," but continues to absorb ethylene until it has reached its capacity. A One Year Refill Kit rounds out the Bluapple ethylene gas management product line, allowing consumers to reuse Bluapples and not add them to landfills.

5.　How to tell if produce is bad and when to toss it? The best way for leafy greens is looking to see if there are any wilted, dark green leaves, and the best way to tell if they have gone south is to smell them. If it smells, it's time to toss it. Fruits are more obvious, since they get soft and/or begin to mold. To learn more about extending the life of produce and the Bluapple product. Visit my website at www.juiceyourwayback.com.

CHAPTER 9

JUICER OR BLENDER: WHICH IS BEST?

I get this question asked so often. What's the best juicer or blender? Both are capable of providing you with a healthy dose of essential vitamins, minerals and enzymes. Although the machines are similar, there is a big difference between these machines. Which one you use depends on what your goals are, whether you have time to cut, peel, and prepare, and how quickly you want to see results.

The key to success to reversing the sign of aging and restoring your health is that you absolutely must get high quality, dense, easily absorbable nutrients in your body, whether this is from juicing or blending makes little difference! In this day and age it's virtually impossible to get adequate nutrition just from eating raw fruits, nuts, and vegetables—even organic ones. However, the fastest way possible, which is with either juicing and/or blending.

Both juicing and blending give you a huge shot of dense nutrition that your body will absorb like a sponge. There are some important differences, but the main thing is that it isn't a contest—both make a valuable contribution to a raw food lifestyle, though in different ways.

Juicers: Juicers extract the juice nutrients from fruits and vegetables and discard the fiber. Juicing provides the body a break from digesting your food, since nutrients are absorbed much more quickly and provide the body with a larger percentage of nutrients then blending. Raw vegetable juices are digested and assimilated within ten to fifteen minutes after we drink them and they are used almost entirely in the nourishment and regeneration of the cells and tissues, glands, and organs of the body. In this case the result is obvious, as the entire process of digestion and assimilation is completed with a maximum degree of speed and efficiency, and with a minimum of effort on the part of the digestive system.

Benefits: Provide relief for those who have sensitive digestive systems that inhibit the digestion of fiber. Juicing delivers a high dose of nutrients and gives your digestive system a rest so it can focus on repairing the body. Juicers provide less heat than blenders, which is important since heat often kills life-giving enzymes.

There are four different types: centrifugal, masticating, twin-gear, and hard-crack juicers.

Drawbacks: Removes all fiber. Fiber is essential in cleansing the body and keeping you feeling full longer. Juicers cost more then blenders. Often you must purchase a lot more produce then you would if you were blending. It also takes more time to cut produce and to clean up.

Blenders: Mixes juice, skin, and fiber together. Just like juicers, blenders come in many different options, from low speed to high speed, with and without pulverizing features. High speed blenders are best to get a consistency near that of a juicer.

Benefits: Blenders cost less than juicers. The fiber retained during blending supports your digestive system by sweeping and eliminating toxins from your digestives system. Blending and/ or smoothies balance out your blood sugar levels since blending raw fruits and vegetables are absorbed much slower in your blood stream than juicing because of the added fiber. Preparation is very fast, and the blender itself is easy to clean.

Drawbacks: Blenders oxidize (age) raw produce, meaning it forces air and heat into the fruits and vegetables causing them to be less potent. Heat kills healthy enzymes. I recommend simply adding ice to your smoothie to minimize this effect. Blending often includes more calories per severing than juicing because fiber is caloric.

Summary:

I've found that having both a juicer and a blender is best, maximizing the benefits of getting fiber in your diet and higher potency of nutrients and enzymes by juicing. My recommendation is buy enough organic produce for a week, and juice half of all the ingredients and freeze the juice in BPA-free ice cube trays, and refrigerate the rest of the produce. As I do quite often is when I want the benefits of both juicing and blending and or when I'm in a rush, I simply take out the juice ice cubes and put a couple of them in a blender with filtered water, then add fresh ingredients and blend. That's a quick, nutrient potent, fiber-filled juice/smoothie in less than two minutes I like to call juice blending.

Freezing juice is also perfect if you don't have a lot of time, or when you run out of fresh produce to blend. Simply pop two or three cubes in a blender with filter water, and you have a healthy juice fast. Juicing for the week saves you a ton of time cutting produce and cleaning the juicer multiple times a day. By adding two to three juice cubes and fresh produce multiple times a day, you will get added fiber and potency of juicing without all the hassle and clean up of using a juicer daily. By combining both juicing and blending you can be on-the-go in less than three minutes. To see a demonstration, go to our website at www.juiceyourwayback.com and click on our YouTube channel.

CHAPTER 10

THE BEST TIME TO JUICE— BODY CYCLES

We all want to lose weight and eat healthier. Did you know that the body has cycles, regular times during which it eliminates waste, and regular times when it assimilates and absorbs the benefits of food? Below, we will outline the best time to juice and the best times to eat food. By learning these cycles, you will arm yourself with knowledge that will help you achieve your goals faster and more effectively.

The Body has Three Cycles

Elimination, Accumulation, and Absorption

4:00 a.m. to Noon (Elimination Cycle). This is the time during which your body eliminates toxins, chemicals, acids, waste, urine, excrement, sweat, and other bodily secretions. In general there are four primary toxin removal systems that must all be working in harmony with one another.

1. The disposal of cellular waste products, especially lactic acid.

2. The removal of larger waste products through your lymphatic system (smaller waste products go into your veins and are exhaled or sent directly to your liver).

3. The processing of toxins by your liver, most of which then goes into the bile ducts and then into your digestive track for final clearance. (Some are made water-soluble and go to your kidneys to be passed in urine.)

4. The final clearance of products by your digestive tract.

5. These four systems tend to flow into one another. One of the

reasons we are sick, tired, and look older then we are is that poor diet, toxic overload and lack of sleep hampers the body's ability to eliminate toxins in this timeframe. It's important to note that we need to get this process up and running again efficiently, and if you are committed in following the steps I've outlined, you will notice a drastic change in your health and appearance.

What to do and what to eat during this process:

From 4am to noon or upon waking you should help the body cleanses by drinking lots of filtered water, apple cider vinegar or lemon juice. After this you should only juice or eat fruit or veggies, best to make a juice or smoothie. For example, blend our recommended smoothies or eat a bowl of in season-fruit. Forty-five minutes before noon, eat, juice, or blend your last meal. You can eat or juice all the juice and veggie blends you want until noon.

By eating and juicing during this time, you are assisting your body's elimination cycle. This helps your body to eliminate toxins and acids form your body and blood. It's these toxins that are preventing you from restoring your health, achieving your weight-loss goals, and looking and feeling younger.

Note: Eating solid foods for breakfast—eggs, potatoes, rice, meat, cereal, milk, and so on—before noon stops the elimination process and interferes with your body's ability to finish its cycle of toxic elimination, and eventually leads to toxic buildup sickness and weight gain. It takes over three hours to digest heavy, starchy, protein-based foods, so the food you eat should be a juice, smoothie, or bowl of fruit to assist your body in effectively eliminating toxic waste.

Noon to 8:00 p.m. (Accumulation Cycle). This is when you should be taking food in and digesting it. Digestion time varies between individuals, and between men and women. After you eat, it takes about six to eight hours for food to pass through your stomach and small intestine. Food then enters your large intestine (colon) for further digestion, absorption of water and, finally, elimination of undigested food. Your body can only digest one solid food at a time. A solid food is one that does not contain 70% water, like fruits and vegetables do, and whose water has been eliminated by cooking, baking or microwaving.

What to do and what to eat during this process:

Your stomach can only work on one solid food at a time, so your lunch, snacks, and dinner must only include one solid food each. Lunch or an in-between snack may include one of the following: chicken, tuna, fish, and always include a green salad or steamed or raw vegetable or green juice. Choose olive oil, vinegar, etc. for salads instead of pre-prepared dressings.

Mixing a protein-heavy meal with carbohydrates causes the stomach to work harder and require different concentrations of digestive juices. This interrupts the elimination cycle, and reduces energy.

Bad Combination Choices:	Good Combination Choices:
protein and rice	meat, salad, veggie, or green juice
protein and noodles	meat, salad, veggie, or green juice
protein and potatoes	meat, salad, veggie, or green juice
protein and cheese, toast, or bread	meat, salad, veggie, or green juice
protein and nuts or beans	meat, salad, veggie, or green juice

It's okay to combine carbs (i.e. rice and potatoes) but avoid pairing a protein with carbohydrates at all costs. That will set the stage for severe illness later in life. A protein requires acid for digestion, and a carbohydrate requires alkaline juices, so this combination produces acid juices and alkaline digestive juices at the same time. It also produces water, which creates digestive juices that cannot fully digest either type of food. Then the body produces more acid and more alkaline juices, which are again neutralized. The cycle continues until the food in your stomach starts to putrefy and ferment, causing gas and acids. The combination of gas and acids leads to acid reflux.

Eating the right combinations of foods helps preserve energy for the elimination cycle, and prevents you from creating spoiled food in your stomach that is converted quickly into acid waste. Remember our goal is to become more alkaline, not acidic. Acid residue from improperly combining foods results in illness and fat storage in our bodies. This is the reason that most people, as they age, come down with various illnesses that terminate their lives early or cause excessive weight gain.

Things to Avoid: It's best to avoid breads, chips or sodas, diet sodas, and excessive water when eating. Excess water or liquids will dilute your digestive acids and slow down digestion of your food. Always choose room temperature water as opposed to cold liquids, as cold liquids will slow the digestive processes. The goal of eating and drinking this way is to free your body from unnecessary energy usage and digestion to better eliminate toxins.

If you want to get the most the benefits from removing toxins and flushing your body, it's best to drink your juice or smoothie on an empty stomach at lease half hour before a meal.

8:00 p.m. to 4:00 a.m. (Absorption Cycle). This is when your body is absorbing and using the food you have eaten during the previous cycle. The role of absorption is vital to the body because, without it, the vitamins, minerals, carbohydrates, and other nutrients we consume cannot be used. Absorption is the process by which the nutrients in food are passed on to the blood. The majority of absorption occurs in the small intestines, the digestive tract's primary organ.

After food passes through the stomach to the small intestines, it is turned into energy for the body to use. Absorption is made possible by the villi, small, bristle-like protrusions in the mucosa. The mucosa is the moist tissue lining certain parts of the body's passages and organs. The villi act as channels through which nutrients can pass into the bloodstream and be carried to the rest of the body. The actual absorption process is slightly different for each type of nutrient.

What to do and what to eat during this process:

Before dinner, you can drink a green juice or smoothie. The important thing is to use organic juice blends in conjunction with the body cycles and properly choose your food combination for optimal health and fitness. This will give you the best results as far as regaining energy and youth, and eliminating disease.

Eat your last meal by 6:00 to 7:00 p.m. so that your food has digested by the time you go to bed. Remember, anything you do differently will disturb these cycles and extend them. When this happens, your food turns into acid, which eventually leads to illness and excessive weight gain, disease, and premature aging.

CHAPTER 11

COMMON JUICING MISTAKES

Juicing is a great way to get nutrients that assist the body in restoring cell regeneration and creating a healthy, youthful glow. By juicing, nutrients are absorbed straight into your bloodstream, giving your body a shot of life giving vitamins, minerals, and enzymes. One of the common mistakes newcomers make when juicing is adding too much fruit into their fresh juices and smoothies. Although fruits are filled with vitamins and minerals, they also expose your body to a large amount of sugar, which spikes insulin levels.

The goal is to add 70-90% of vegetables, with the remainder being fruits to give your juice or blend a boost of sweetness and flavor. Too much fructose (fruit sugars) cause your blood sugar levels to spike, which is good for sustaining energy levels and very bad for the large percentage of Americans that carry parasites in their gut, or have diabetes.

If you have a tough time at 70-90% vegetables, try adding lemon or lime in to cut the bitter flavor, since these are low in sugar and high in flavor.

Timing is Everything

If you want to get the most benefits from removing toxins and flushing your body, it's best to drink your juice or smoothie on an empty stomach at least half an hour before a meal. Your body will be able to absorb all the nutrients of the juice or smoothie quicker and use the minimal amount of digestive energy in the process.

When using juicing to restore your youthful appearance, juicing is not meant to be a meal replacement. Think of it as taking the best vitamins on the planet.

Sip Your Juice or Smoothie

Juice is not meant to be drunk in one gulp like a shot of tequila. Enjoy the flavor, and take your time. Swirling it around in your month before your swallow boosts digestive enzymes that help your body digest your juice much faster. Our stomach and digestive system are very sensitive. If you gulp a juice or smoothie down on the run, your body is in a state of flight or flight and will compromise the digestive process and uptake of nutrients.

Drink Your Juice Right Away

Try to drink your juice or smoothie right away. After ten to twenty minutes, light and air will destroy a large percentage of the nutrients, and antioxidants will loose their potency. If you must store your juice, transfer to a dark, airtight, non-BPA container or ice cube tray and put it in the fridge or freezer. If in the fridge, consume it within twenty-four hours. It may not be as nutrient-dense as fresh juice, but it's still better than not drinking juice at all.

CHAPTER 12

AGE-REVERSING JUICE BLENDS

The goal is of reversing premature aging and restoring your natural healthy glow is to eliminate toxins and flood your cells with processed free, organic fruits, vegetables, and herbs. The list below has some of the most effective superfoods that boost immunity cells and nourish, replenish, and rebuild the body from the inside out.

The anti-aging fruits, vegetables, and herbs below do not have measurements of ingredients to blend or juice. Don't get hung up on that. Consistency is what will restore your health and reverse or stop aging in its tracks. Again, if you are taking any medications, please consult with a doctor about any possible adverse reactions these ingredients may have with any medications you're taking.

The idea of including the anti-aging benefits of each ingredient is to educate you on the how the ingredient helps your body restore and rebuild from the inside out. While working with many clients, I've found that people's tastes are different; by including a robust list of known anti-aging ingredients, I've given you the power to mix and match ingredients to your specific goals and taste.

As mentioned, we mostly age on a cellular level from the inside out, meaning that the amount of toxins you eat, drink, or smoke can either make your skin glow, or look old and wrinkled. No longer do you need fancy, overpriced creams, lotions, cleansers, or serums to nourish your skin. While genetics, the environment, and other lifestyle choices play a role in your skin's appearance, don't underestimate the power of anti-aging superfoods when it comes to turning back the appearance of age and puffy dark circles.

Deficiencies in minerals like zinc and selenium have been linked to acne and dull-looking skin.

The radiance of our hair, skin, and nails in part depends on how "mineralized" we are. To combat unhealthy, depleted skin, we need to nourish our bodies with anti-oxidant-rich superfoods. Below are some examples of the most powerful foods you can consume to reverse age and cause your skin to become radiant. Again, it is my recommendation that before you blend these anti-aging superfoods you must of completed the toxic elimination process of identifying toxins in your life and removing them from food to products (2-6 weeks) and have started a cycle of acid resistant probiotics supplements or superfoods.

Instructions

Blend or juice a minimum of five to six of the ingredients below in one to two juices or smoothies per day. If juicing, remember you will need a lot of the ingredients to get a glass or two of juice, whereas blending doesn't require as many ingredients. It's also a great idea to juice larger amounts of ingredients and freeze them in ice cube trays so you can juice and blend faster during the week without as much prep and clean up. See chapter 14 for additional benefits on juicing and blending on-the-go and in under five minutes. Always wash all ingredients and choose in-season, organic produce when available. Use our list of what ingredients you must buy organic, and those that you don't need to buy organic in chapter seven.

Watercress – Considered one of the highest density, most nutrient-rich foods on the plant, watercress contains more Vitamin C than oranges, and four times more beta carotene and vitamin A than tomatoes or broccoli. These essential vitamins are proven to improve skin conditions and reduce wrinkles. Watercress purifies the blood and keeps you free from skin inflammation and infections. Eating, blending, or juicing this herb daily increases energy and improves skin conditions such as acne, redness, and rosacea.

Apples – An apple a day keeps the doctor away, but it keeps wrinkles away as well. In addition to vitamin C, apples are a good source of quercetin, which is a potent antioxidant that helps fight free-radical damage in skin cells. The molecular structure of quercetin is extremely well-suited for destroying free radicals, which makes it an excellent wrinkle fighter. When buying apples, choose organically grown apples if possible. Apples contain the highest levels of pesticides and other chemicals when conventionally grown.

Celery – Celery contains Vitamin K, which helps to reduce high blood pressure. This can reduce your stress level. Stress can cause bad skin, migraines, even cancer. Celery also contains natural sodium, potassium and water, and can help to prevent dehydration. Dehydrated skin means dryness, flaking, wrinkles, and even breakouts. Juice or blend celery every day or at least every other day. When buying celery, choose organically grown produce. Celery tops the list of vegetables that contain the highest levels of neurotoxin pesticides and chlorothalonil, which is believed to be carcinogenic.

Kale – A superfood powerhouse loaded with antioxidants, which help your body fight the harmful effects of oxidation. Many health problems stem from the effects of oxygen on the body. When oxygen is metabolized, it creates free radicals. This process accelerates aging, converts healthy cells into cancerous ones, elevates blood pressure, hardens arteries, and promotes inflammation and arthritis. Kale helps counter these effects and neutralizes free radicals, and is also a great source of iron, calcium, and vitamins A, C, and K. Kale also has a surprising amount of omega-3 fatty acids, which are an important component of any anti aging diet.

Grapefruit – Slows cell aging and contains large quantities of spermdine. The compound helps cells grow and mature. Spermdine slows aging by inducing autophagy, a process that helps our cells regenerate. The pink pigment found in grapefruit is the presence of lycopene, a powerful antioxidant that combats the body's cell aging effect triggered by free radicals. **Warning:** check with your doctor when juicing or eating grapefruit, because grapefruit binds to enzymes naturally found in your intestine and may affect some medications such as statins, anti-depressants, and calcium blockers.

Strawberries – Contain large amounts of Vitamin C, which plays a role in improving the skin's elasticity and resilience. Vitamin C is also good for collagen formation, which tones and tightens skin. Due to the excellent benefits of vitamin C for skin, it is used in many face washes and skin creams. The heavy amounts of vitamin C helps in anti-aging, prevents wrinkles, acne, blackheads, and blemishes. Strawberries contain ellagic acid, which prevents collagen from breaking and helps to maintain younger-looking skin. Strawberries are also known to reduce joint pain from arthritis.

Blueberries – This fruit is considered one of the top superfoods of all time for its anti-aging benefits. Due to their high concentration of anthocyanin, blueberries contribute to collagen strength by neutralizing enzymes that destroy connective tissue and by scavenging free radicals. The anthocyanin also enhances the effects of the blueberries' vitamin C. Furthermore, compared to other berries, blueberries (especially wild blueberries) are a good source of vitamin E.

Beets – rich in vitamins and minerals, vitamin A and C, folate, fiber, manganese, and potassium. They are filled with antioxidants that revive the skin by eliminating dead cells. They support the liver to increase detoxification, which helps in slowing down the aging process. The nitrates present in beet roots ensure easy blood flow to the brain.

Cucumbers – filled with silicon, which is a mineral essential for building connective tissue. Adding silicon to the diet will give you amazing results in your hair, skin, and nails. Use the whole cucumber as it is, without peeling. Most of the silicon in cucumber is found in the skin itself. They help to improve your hair and nail strength, and control cholesterol levels. They are a good remedy for improved complexion and reducing signs of age.

Avocados – an anti-aging superfood. They are full of vitamin E, potassium, antioxidants, and monounsaturated fat. All of these nutrients are vital for anti-aging efforts. Omega-3s are good fats, which help to maintain cellular integrity. Avocados are excellent for the skin and nails. Instead of juicing or blending, it's recommended you eat avocados daily, in between meals as snacks.

Pineapple – Pineapples are another anti-aging superfood. They are loaded with powerful vitamins and enzymes, which helps reduce the signs of wrinkles. Pineapple is mostly water, but it also includes essential iron, zinc, copper, vitamin B1, B2, B12, C, carotene, potassium, calcium, magnesium, iodine, and manganese. All help reduce inflammation and clear and moisturize the skin. Whether you choose to eat, juice, or apply to your face, pineapple is a power-packed anti-aging fruit. Pineapple's other powerful element is bromelain, which is a composition of enzymes that reduces inflammation and redness on the skin. Bromelain is responsible for most of pineapple's anti-aging benefits.

Turmeric – This vibrant yellow spice, commonly seen in curry, has a wealth of benefits. Among them is the ability to potentially ward off irritants that cause degenerative disease. Turmeric may also reduce oxidative stress. This means it could protect tissues from damage and could be beneficial at preventing wrinkles, scars, and other visible signs of aging.

Red Peppers – help to form collagen and the structural fiber needed to keep skin tight and healthy. Did you know that green peppers are unripe red peppers? Green peppers have half the vitamin C and 1/10 the Vitamin A compared to a ripe red pepper. Red peppers contain 300% of your recommended daily allowance of vitamin C. Red peppers are a great source of vitamin A, B6, and magnesium, and are shown to decrease anxiety, improve the quality of sperm and libido, and build collagen.

Goji Berries – High in antioxidants and amino acids, goji berries increase growth hormone levels, which helps replace old skin. Goji berries help fill in fine lines, smooth skin, and improve skin tone and color. They are high in Vitamin C, which supports the production of collagen, speeds healing, and protects the skin from free radical damage. This amazing fruit has been also shown to help age spots and increase adenosine triphosphate (ATP) by as much as 20%, aiding in the skin's ability to heal.

Raw Cacao – promotes cell repair and rejuvenation, and helps protect and increase blood flow to the skin. Raw cacao can be found in most health food stores. It contains more than 320 antioxidants, the most powerful ingredient to boost collagen protection. The level of antioxidants in the body is directly connected to our biological age and life expectancy. The incredible powers of cacao beans can slow down the aging process significantly, strengthen your immunity, and relieve anxiety, depression, and fatigue.

Parsnips – contain essential nutrients and minerals that help fight aging. Parsnips look like carrots and contain both sugar and starch, which make it very tasty and rich in fiber. Parsnips also contain vitamin C, which helps repair skin cells. Moreover, parsnips help your body's immune system. They work wonders for hair, skin, and nails, too.

Carrots – are good for the eyes and provide essential nutrients for rejuvenation of cells and wrinkle reduction. That's because they're high in beta-carotene, a plant pigment that gives carrots its distinctive color. When consumed, beta-carotene is converted into vitamin A, which then helps your body make new cells to replace the old ones—especially the cells of your skin, eyes, and bones. Only buy organic carrots, for they are amongst the most contaminated with chemicals when conventionally grown.

Kiwis – By now you should understand that vitamin C is a very beneficial vitamin as far as keeping your skin, nails, and hair healthy, youthful, and vibrant. Kiwis offer 137.2 milligrams of vitamin C per serving. Kiwis offer a long list of health and skin benefits such as protection against UV damage, rejuvenation, hydration, and softening of the skin. One study showed that kiwi can help you achieve a radiance much like a tan in just a few weeks of eating, juicing, or blended this power-packed fruit.

Chia Seeds or Flax Seeds – These seeds are loaded with omega-3 fatty acids, proteins and fiber. These three nutrients promote strength, radiance, and a glowing complexion. Omega-3s are known to be powerful anti-inflammatory agent—this is highly effective in reducing joint pain and helping to reduce or eliminate dark puffiness under the eyes.

Sulfur - The third most abundant mineral in your body, sulfur is known to be the single most effective compound at reducing winkles. It is present in every cell, but is concentrated most strongly in the hair, skin, and nails. It helps your body function, playing an important role in your body's electron transport system, proper vitamin conversion, detoxification, joint health, and proper insulin function. It also helps promote circulation and decrease inflammation. Sulfur must also be present for the body to produce collagen, which keeps skin soft and supple. You can see why it is often referred to as the "healing mineral" or the "beauty mineral!"

For maximum health benefits, it is best to obtain sulfur through your diet. The primary dietary sources of sulfur are fish, grass-fed beef, and free-range poultry. It's also available in the foods below, albeit in lesser amounts.

Foods High in Sulfur

- Broccoli
- Cabbage
- Cauliflower
- Garlic
- Kale
- Onions
- Asparagus
- Brussels sprouts
- Apple seed oil
- Leeks
- Shallots
- Chives

Topical use of sulfur has great benefits as well. Skin and hair issues (like psoriasis, eczema, acne and dandruff) have been treated with sulfur-containing compounds and waters for centuries. Hippocrates, the father of modern medicine, used sulfur preparations to treat skin conditions. And the ancient Romans soaked themselves in sulfuric waters to treat skin problems, relieve pain, and to prevent aging. Sulfur is a keratolytic agent, which means that it helps to shed dead skin cells. Dead skin cells are responsible for blocking pores and creating the conditions necessary for the multiplication of acne-causing bacteria, eczema, and psoriasis. Sulfur also helps to clarify the skin, banish excess oil, minimize pores, and helps prevent and heal blemishes. It is an excellent solution for breakouts on the chest, back, and face. This is just one of the reasons why we included cold-pressed apple seed oil, a natural, rich, whole-food source of sulfur.

CHAPTER 13

SKIN PROBLEM JUICE RECIPES

If you have skin problems and want to enhance your appearance, or have smooth skin that is blemish free, stop wasting your money on expensive, chemically toxic cosmetics and consider the juicing recipes below. Organic raw juices can have unbelievable effects on your skin tone and texture. Keep in mind that none of these recipes below will work overnight—but if you want to have perfect skin, more energy, and feel and look younger, the long-term way to achieve this is not by using drugs, Botox, or plastic surgery. These methods are treating the symptoms of premature aging, and not curing the root cause of wrinkles and problem skin, which is malnutrition of skin cells and of your immune system. You must remember it's about identifying and eliminating chemicals and toxins from your daily routine, and nourishing your skin cells from the inside out with plant-based foods and chemical-free products.

Acne

This chronic, inflammatory affliction is also called blackheads, whiteheads, and pimples. Acne is affected by diet, which is often loaded with fat, grease, and sugar—all very toxic. The result is an acidic buildup in the blood, leaving the body no choice but to deposit these toxins in the largest organ in your body, your skin. This condition is often treated with creams and ointments, some of which actually burn your skin and irritate it further.

First, you must make the choice to eliminate fried food and foods which are high in trans-fatty acids, such as milk, margarine, and vegetable oils. Instead, incorporate the superfoods discussed here.

Clear Skin Recipe
- Spinach
- Carrots
- Green apple
- Parsley

Optional add 1/2 cup of ice and water if blending.

Dry Skin

Red, itchy, flaky skin is unsightly and annoying. While it neither life-threatening nor a skin disease, it can be dramatically reduced by drinking fresh organic vegetable juice. Cucumbers are best for their powerful effectiveness as a diuretic. By flushing out the chemical toxins in your body and accumulated waste materials, a healthy glow is restored to the skin. Cucumbers have potassium and phosphorus, both of which help restore vitality not only to damaged skin, but to nails and hair as well.

Rehydration Recipe
- Tomato
- Cucumber
- Celery
- 2 cloves or garlic if juicing/1 if blending
- Parsley

Optional: add 1/2 cup of ice and water if blending.

Psoriasis

This chronic skin disease is characterized by red patches, which are covered with white scales. Its occurs when skin cells divide too quickly—up to a thousand times faster than normal cell division. It usually occurs on the scalp, buttocks, wrists, elbows, knees and feet. Almost anything can cause it, especially stress or a weak immune system due to lack of proper nutrition.

Eat foods high in fiber that bind to toxins and help move them out of the body. Eliminate alcohol and eat cold-water fatty fish, like mackerel, salmon, sardines and herring.

As with eczema, the best relief comes from celery juice, which is high in sodium and magnesium. It's hard on the liver, but mix with Swiss chard, cucumber, and carrots, and it's easy to metabolize and has a pleasant taste.

- Cucumbers
- Celery
- Carrots
- Parsley
- Celery

Optional: add 1/2 cup of ice and water if blending.

Wrinkles

As we age, our skin loses it elasticity, and telomeres—the strands at the end of chromosomes—shorten. As we age, feeding our bodies chemicals and toxins, telomeres shorten and cause the skin cells to weaken and sag. However, one of the best ways to slow down the process of premature telomere shortening is to quit smoking, get plenty of sleep (seven to eight hours a night), go to bed before 10:00 p.m., drink plenty of water, and follow the detox programs and recipes above. Reduce all foods made with saturated fats, fast foods, junk foods, starches, and give up sugary drinks and alcohol. Instead, load up on healthy, high-fiber foods with plenty of fresh fruits and green vegetables, including cucumbers.

One of the greatest vegetables to hydrate and nourish the skin and help minimize wrinkles is cucumbers. These green veggies are the world's best rejuvenators for hydration and improving one's skin. It flushes old waste and chemical toxins from the blood and helps the skin glow. This blend is sure give your skin that glow and suppleness associated with younger-looking skin.

Skin Rejuvenator

- Cucumbers
- Parsley
- Spinach
- Beets

Optional: add 1/2 cup of ice and water if blending.

CHAPTER 14

JUICING IN UNDER FIVE MINUTES AND ON-THE-GO

With our busy, hectic lives, people often tell me they don't have the time to prepare, cut, and juice. It's one of the major reasons so many of us choose processed or fast foods these days..

In this chapter I will teach you how to minimize the time it takes to cut, prepare, and juice at home and on the run. You will learn timesaving tips and tricks to juice in five minutes or less.

Juicing is a better option to achieve faster results for your body. However, juicing takes more time to prepare, juice, and clean up than blending. However, fiber from blending is very beneficial in cleansing and eliminating age-robbing toxins. After experimenting for several years, I've learned the fastest way to get the nutrient-dense vitamins and minerals from juicing, and combine it with the fiber-rich benefits and ease of clean up of blending, is something I call juice blending.

Juice Blending

You will need to have a juicer and either a blender or extractor, and up to 4 BPA-free ice cube trays or glass mason jars. Since most fruits and vegetables lose up to 50% of their nutrients, vitamins, and enzymes between the time they are picked and when they arrive on your table, it's imperative that you purchase all your organic produce at once and juice them as quickly as possible.

Step 1. Pick a day where you will have about one to two hours to shop, juice, and clean up. Once you return home from your trip to the grocery store, pull out your juicer and juice the recommended ingredients according to what you want to achieve, from cleansing to rejuvenation. Don't get hung up on the measurements and/or portions of each ingredient; the goal is to be consistent and incorporate a juice blend one to three times a day.

Step 2. After you've juiced all the ingredients, mix the juice before you pour it into an ice cube trays or glass mason jars. Carefully place into the freezer. Depending on how often you will be juice blending, you may want to cover the juice trays with plastic wrap or purchase BPA-free ice cube trays with lids—or simply use mason jars. Don't worry about covering them if you will be juicing frequently.

Step 3. Before your first juice blend, make sure to drink your full two to three glasses of water upon waking to assist the body in finishing the elimination of toxins. After about an hour, you are ready to juice blend.

Simply place two to three juice cubes in your blender/extractor and add some fresh veggies and fruit to your juice cubes and blend.

Juice Blending Benefits

- By juice blending, you get both the higher concentration of nutrients from juicing and the fiber and convenience of blending. Fiber is a cleansing agent that assists the body in elimination of toxins, and scraps and cleans the lining of the digestive system, which is responsible for assimilating nutrients into the body. Fiber also helps you feel full longer than juicing alone.
- Since green vegetables and some fruits keep longer, like spinach, apples, kale, Brussels sprouts, broccoli, carrots, etc., make sure you have some on hand to add to your juice cubes when blending for the healthy fiber and extra vitamins.

- By freezing your juice, it will keep longer. A large percentage of nutrients are lost in the trip from farm to table. By juicing your produce on the day of purchase, you preserve nutrients that would otherwise be lost from sitting in your refrigerator until you're ready to juice.

- Using glass jars or BPA-free containers and freezing, you can bring your juice on the road. It takes about two hours at room temperature to defrost and four to six hours in the refrigerator.

- Clean up and convenience. By juicing one day a week and juice blending the remainder of the week, you can juice in less than two to five minutes. In addition, the clean up is a simple rinse or wash.

CHAPTER 15

ANTI-AGING EXERCISES

Scientists have discovered that regular exercise may be the key to reversing the skin's aging process. Researchers at McMaster University in Ontario found that those who started working out later in life could achieve younger-looking skin from working out. Exercising is one of the best youth serums in the arsenal you have to fight premature aging. Your level of fitness affects how youthful you look, the ease with which you move, and your ability to fight off disease and reverse the signs of aging.

Below are some simple exercises you can do either at the gym or on-the-go. No matter how old you are or what you like to do for exercise, you can incorporate the below exercises into your routine to move better, protect yourself from injury, and look and feel younger.

1. Re-program your genetics

Ever hear that you can't change your genes? That's only partially true. While you can't change your genetic makeup, you can change how certain genes are expressed—that is, how much they do whatever they do. And strength training is one of the best ways to do that. Only twenty-six weeks of resistance training reverses the aging process at the genetic level, research shows. "You can actually train your tissues to behave the way they did when you were younger," Hagan says. Furthermore, resistance training preserves muscle mass that we typically lose as we age—five pounds per decade, on average. (We also gain an average of ten pounds of fat per decade. "That's certainly not fair! It should at least be even!" Hagan says. Agreed!)

2. Do more cardio than you think you need

While U.S. guidelines call for 150 minutes of cardio per week, Hagan's examination of research found that 240 minutes per week is optimal for heart health. Aerobic activity improves mitochondrial function (the work of energy-producing organelles in cells), which typically decreases with age. Do four hours of cardio a week sound like too much? "If you don't have much time, interval training is one of the most efficient ways to exercise at high enough levels to improve aerobic fitness," Hagan says.

3. Make your two brains talk to each other

Include some moves where you cross your legs and arms over the midline of your body. Why? The connection between the right and left hemispheres of your brain deteriorates as you age, which causes "brain farts" (technical name: brain delays) as the hemispheres begin to have trouble communicating with one another, Hagan explains. Crossing limbs forces the two sides of your brain to talk to one another, strengthening the connection between hemispheres. How cool is that?

4. Embrace high-impact activity

A lot of older people are afraid to jump because it'll hurt their knees and hips. "But that's bogus, because you need to jump in everyday life, and you need impact to build bone density," Hagan says. That doesn't mean you need to take up Insanity (the DVD series known for crazy-intense jumping moves). A "forceful step," like you're squishing a bug, is enough of an impact to make a difference. Think of forceful stepping any time you lunge, squat, or march.

5. Walk the Age Away

The average American walks only 2,000 steps per day, but experts recommend 10,000. "7,500 steps a day is what we Canadians call the BAM, or bare you-know-what minimum, for health," Hagan says. Studies show that merely tracking your steps doubles how many you take, so strap on a step meter and see if you can beat your count every day.

Don't Have Time to Exercise – Try These Simple Steps

Who has time these days to join a gym, drive there, work out, and come home make dinner, pick up the kids, clean, etc., etc. Don't get me wrong; exercise is essential to reverse aging, but there are things you can do to save time and money that are just as effective as joining a gym, and you can easily incorporate them into your daily routine.

You can burn off the same number of calories (or more), as you would by spending an hour at gym or in an aerobics' class with these simple steps. It's so easy. In fact, you probably did some of these today, and you didn't even know it. Let me explain.

Remember the days when we had to walk into the gas station to pay? When you mowed your own lawn? Or back in the day, when you had to get off the couch to change the channel on your TV? These are just a few of the tasks that are becoming obsolete, depriving us of physical activity. If you add up all the extra calories you could have burned just from doing a few things that involve actually moving, you could reverse the aging process, increase your energy, and lose up to thirty pounds a year! Hard to believe, but it's true. Most of the activities we used to do are being replaced by technology, making it much easier to gain weight, have weight-related diseases, and look much older then we are.

If you have free time to drive to the gym, work out, go for a run, or take long walks, or bike rides, or any other form of physical exercise—that's great. But let's be realistic: most of us have very little free time.

There's no doubt that regular physical activity three or more times a week can help:

- Control your weight
- Decrease stress
- Evaluates better mood
- Enhances memory
- Jump start your sex drive
- Improve sleep quality
- Slow cell aging
- Keep your skin soft and glowing
- Improve posture
- Lower your risk of heart disease
- Lower your risk for type 2 diabetes and metabolic syndrome
- Lower your risk of some cancers
- Strengthen your bones and muscles
- Improve your ability to do daily activities and prevent falls, if you're an older adult
- Increase your chances of living longer

The good news is that by adding our juice recipes into your daily diet as well as adding simple activities back into your daily life, you can shape up, burns calories, and look and feel younger in just thirty days.

A recent Cooper Institute study found that lifestyle activities such as climbing stairs and parking your car in the farthest space offer benefits similar to those gained in a gym workout. In fact, exercise doesn't just make you feel younger—it may actually turn off the aging process in your chromosomes. It has to do with telomeres, which become shorter as you get older. Longer telomeres are associated with longevity. According to a study from UCSF, a link was found between regular exercise and the lengthening of the telomeres, suggesting that exercise can slow aging. "Though exercise won't guarantee you a long life and looking ten to twenty years younger, it can greatly improve your odds," says Frisch.

Here are eight simple ways to bump up your activity level—and burn calories and look and feel younger.

1. Speed Up. Increase the intensity of your everyday tasks, from vacuuming to walking. Increasing your speed in every task can burn an extra fifteen calories, and increase your heart rate and overall health. Turn on some music, add in some vigorous bursts, and enjoy the movement to burn more calories and have fun.

2. Take Stairs. Climbing stairs is a great leg strengthener, because you're lifting your body weight against gravity. In addition to taking the stairs at every opportunity, try stepping up and down on the curb while you're waiting for the bus, at the bank, or filling your gas tank. Also try taking the steps two at a time when using the stairs. It's a great way to build and shape your buttocks.

3. Flex. Although some people believe that you must workout vigorously to burn calories, a movement as small as flexing your muscles can also burn calories. This is because calories are energy, so anything that uses energy burns calories. Squeezing your muscles throughout the day can considerably increase the calories you burn. Tighten your butt, abs, and/or stomach at every red light, or while driving or watching TV.

4. Think of bags as dumbbells. When you let someone else load your groceries or carry your suitcase, you're missing a great opportunity for strengthening and calorie burning, says certified coach Beth Rothenberg, who teaches a class for fitness professionals at UCLA.

"Carry your groceries, balanced with a bag in each hand, even if you have to make several trips," she says. "And pack two smaller suitcases instead of one big one, so you can carry them yourself."

5. Have a ball. Replace your desk chair with a giant exercise ball, says Cedric X. Bryant, PhD, chief exercise physiologist for the American Council on Exercise in San Diego, where many staffers have adopted this idea. "You have to engage the core muscles to maintain stability," he says, "so you're getting a great workout right at your desk."

6. Go the distance. "Stop using the closest restroom, parking space, or vending machine," says Minneapolis fitness trainer Sandra Swami. As the instructor of a program that's designed to help working women get more active, Swami urges her clients to get in the habit of taking the longest route to the rest room (on a different floor, if that's possible) and to climb stairs to get there.

7. Air Squats. Next time you're taking a shower, brushing your teeth, or watching TV, simply squat. Air squats engage your legs and butt muscles; they also work your core, back, and shoulders, increase mobility, and lift and shape the legs and buttocks.

Things to remember when attempting an air squat:

- Keep your weight on your heels.
- Keep your torso upright with your shoulders pulled back.
- Your feet should be hip-width apart with your toes slightly pointing outward.
- Your knees should be over (but not beyond) your toes.
- Your butt, back, and core muscles should be engaged the entire time.
- Raise your arms while squatting down and bring them back to your side on the way up, keeping your shoulders

back. This helps with balancing yourself.

- On the downward portion of the squat, aim to go *below* parallel.

Do them often, and you'll soon be an air-squat-juice-your-way-back master!

8. Play waiting games. Don't just sit there while your computer is downloading, or the copier is collating. Do a stretch (place both hands behind your head, open your elbows, and lean back), try balancing on one leg, or do a few buttocks squeezes.

Also try these simple steps to increase physical activity:

- Fire your gardener if you have one—do it yourself - **400 calories.**
- Wash your own car – **282 calories.**
- Fire your maid – do it yourself – **152 calories.**
- Play a round of golf – without a cart - **721 calories (9 holes).**
- Focus on walking faster then you normally do – **15 extra calories.**
- Walk up escalators, never just stand or ride one again – Works legs and buttocks.
- When at work and no one is around, do squats – Works legs and buttocks.
- When at home, do squats in front of the TV – Works legs and buttocks.
- When sitting down at work do calf raises – Works calf muscles and circulation.
- Go for a swim, walk, bike ride, hula hoop with kids, or take up an outdoor activity.

Fitting regular exercise into your daily schedule may seem difficult at first, but even ten minutes at a time is fine. The key is to find the right exercise for you. It should be fun and match your abilities.

CHAPTER 16

TIPS ON HOW TO LOOK YOUNGER

Turn in Earlier

Going to bed by 10:00 p.m. is one the best things you can do to get the regenerative sleep required to rebuild cells and eliminate toxins. If you go to bed around 10:00 p.m., your body goes through a transformation process, releasing and raising levels of melatonin production. It is also known that if you miss this window at the beginning of your sleep cycle, it will take you much longer to typically fall asleep. The quality of that sleep will also be less, and you'll feel a sense of fatigue in the morning.

Adjusting your bedtime from, say, midnight to 10:00 p.m. will have a huge impact on the quality of your sleep. The reason for this is that you are taking advantage of our natural biological sleep process, which starts around 10:00 p.m. If you're going to bed much later than this, try to shorten this by ten to fifteen minutes a night until you're closer to the ideal sleep cycle.

If you are having trouble falling asleep or suffer from insomnia, there are several things you can do reset your off beat sleep cycle;

1. Don't watch TV or work on a computer later than 9:00 p.m., the earlier the better. Both of these activities stimulate the mind and trick your body thinking it's daylight, thus suppressing the sleep cycle.

2. Remove any TVs or computers from your bedroom. Minimize your bedroom activities to sleep, relaxation, and making love, not

working or worrying. Make your bedroom your meditation zone for relaxing and reflecting on all the great things in your life.

3. Stop drinking caffeinated drinks. Even drinking caffeine in the morning affects your ability to fall asleep at night, because over time it causes a chemical shift towards being awake and affects your natural sleep cycles.

4. Eat a smaller dinner. You know by now that eating later in the day your digestion system gets weaker. Eating a large dinner at night or past 8:00 p.m. interrupts your ability to fall asleep because your body is contending between winding down and ramping up the digestive process.

5. Avoid naps during the day until you can fall asleep by 10:00 p.m.

6. If you often get up at night to urinate, don't drink liquids after 7:00 p.m. The kidneys typically process liquids in ninety minutes.

Power of Belief

One of our most overlooked superpowers in life is the power of our beliefs. What is a belief? The dictionary defines it as: 1. A state or habit of mind in which trust or confidence is placed in some person or thing. 2. Conviction of the truth of some statement or the reality of some being or phenomenon, especially when based on examination of evidence. A belief is something that *we personally choose* to form in our own minds about the way *we choose* to perceive the world around us. It is our recognition that some idea or thing is true and valid.

In my opinion, our power of belief is our subconscious mind, listening to our conscious mind and believing it to be true. I see and hear so many stories of failure and success, and what your subconscious believes will often become reality. If you are convinced of something, it becomes your belief. For example, I always get a cold in winter; I always live paycheck-to-paycheck, etc. etc. Did you know that Elvis Presley and Michael Jackson always thought that they would die young? Once you're convinced of something and truly believe in it, your subconscious mind takes steps to ensure it happens. As in the case of Elvis and Michael, who lived a lifestyle that would deliver the results of their beliefs. I have friends that believe they always make lots of money, and guess what they do?

The power of belief is more powerful than most medicines, and promotes rapid healing often without medicine. This is called the placebo effect. Also called the placebo response. A remarkable phenomenon in which a placebo—a fake treatment, an inactive substance like sugar, distilled water, or saline solution—can sometimes improve a patient's condition simply because the person has the expectation that it will be helpful. For example, if you truly believe that eating McDonald's everyday will cause you to lose weight, you will lose weight—but you might not be very healthy. Your brain is the most powerful organ in the universe, and whatever you believe, your body follows.

The one thing you will certainly experience with the *Juice Your Way Back* challenge is that after you eliminate toxins, your brain chemistry will change, and every time you juice you will feel things start to happen. After you finish your smoothie or juice, you will think and feel instantly healthier, even though it takes time to see the results from toxic elimination and juicing.

Again, our beliefs are things that *we decide we want to think are true,* based on the information we have at this point in our lives. Our beliefs are based off of our *perception* of life, which is based solely on our experiences and knowledge. Just because we see something a certain way does not necessarily mean that's the way it actually is.

Perception and reality are two different things. As we get older and learn new things, we realize that certain assumptions we used to have were not as accurate as the view we currently have of the world. This is why I consider myself a student of life—because I know that everything I think I know about the world is just based on the best assumptions I can make, using all of the things I've learned up to this point. That does not necessarily make any of them true.

So if you don't think you deserve to look younger, achieve the body you want, have a super immune system, a better job, a rewarding career, or a successful business, how can you achieve it? How can you reach something if you don't feel you can ever have it?

Instead of complaining about what you don't have, think about all the things you do have and what you want to accomplish. Do you want to look and feel younger, lose weight, get a new job, return to school, or start a business? What steps are you taking to make those things happen?

1. Write down your ideas for the future and talk yourself into it. If you want to look younger, think all day long how much younger you are looking and that your body is amazing at reversing or slowing down the aging process and disease. You first have to talk yourself into it, believe it, and let the subconscious take over. It's that simple! Don't get me wrong—you can't just think about it and it happens—you must be convinced it has already happened and your subconscious will make it happen. Once your subconscious is on board, it will create conscious thoughts and actions that make it happen. When I call a friend of mine and ask how his day is going, he says "I'm a money making machine!" Guess what he believes without question? Once you believe something to be true without a doubt, it happens, and your subconscious leads you do the things necessary to back up your belief.

2. Look at where you are now. Write down the things you'll

need to move forward. For instance, will you need a large investment of money to begin your business? Is specialized training required for that new job or career?

3. Consider your everyday thoughts. Do you go from believing you can reach your goals to being discouraged? If you are always thinking negative thoughts, how can you create a positive life for yourself? What you tell yourself every day does have an impact on your belief system and what happens in your life.

You won't be able to move forward if you don't believe that you can. If you want to make positive and powerful changes, then you have to believe that those changes are possible, without question. You have to be there on the inside long before you see the outside results.

As you start your *Juice Your Way Back* journey, you will start to feel and look better. Your energy level, attitude, and appearance will improve as you get further along in the program. Friends, family and coworkers will notice and ask what's different. As you become knowledgeable about toxin elimination and nutrition, others will want to learn what you're doing. You will start to become a role model, and many will be inspired by you and want to set out on their own journey. As a nutritionist, many of my friends and family members also share my passion for wanting to feel and look better. You too will inspire others and cause a movement of health and fitness. This is perhaps the best benefit you will receive from living the principles of *Juice Your Way Back*; you'll help and inspire others to look and be healthier. They say the true meaning of success is to know that one life has breathed easier because you have existed. It is my hope that you too will be successful in sharing the knowledge you learned here to inspire others to live and breath easier. God bless and live well.

CHAPTER 17

QUESTIONS AND ANSWERS

Q. Do I have to detox before I start the anti-aging blends?

A. Yes. For many years, your body has been layering fecal matter and chemical toxic particles, coating your small intestines in a substance called ileum, which prevents you from absorbing nutrients. If this is not cleansed, you'll be wasting your time and money.

Q. How strict a diet must I follow?

A. Once you remove most of the parasites and toxins from your body, the organs and metabolism will most likely return to full capacity. The goal of toxin elimination and balancing out your good bacteria is to put your body in balance. I believe in rewards for hard work and use an 80/20 rule. 80-90% organic, non-toxic processed foods, and meats. 10-20% foods that you love once in a while, as a reward. If ice cream is your thing, simply choose organic and enjoy without feeling guilty. Processed foods may make you sick after you have purified your body, but the key is to reward yourself once in a while and enjoy life.

Q. Do I really need to drink lots of water when I wake?

A. Yes! This is critical in assisting the body in the final stage of waste and toxin elimination. Side effects will be better skin, more energy, and weight loss. Never drink unfiltered water.

Q. How times must I juice or blend per day?

A. The ideal answer is twice per day. Once in the morning, after your two to four glasses of water or organic apple cider vinegar with the mothers. And once in the afternoon, when you get home from work or before you eat dinner. Juicing before you eat dinner helps digestion and fills you up.

Q. Must I only eat or juice organic?

A. The goal is to reduce the body's toxin overload so that it can eliminate toxins and waste. Otherwise toxins, hormones, pesticides, chemicals, and any antibiotics you consume will be stored in your body. For meats and fish—definitely eat only organic. For fruits and vegetables and nuts, refer to the chapter on what you need to buy organic and what you can buy non-organic.

Q. How quickly will I start to see and feel results?

A. Once you start, you may experience negative side effects. Think of this as withdrawal. This is normal. After about a week you should start having more energy and feeling better every day. Once you're through the detox section of the program and start flooding your cells with anti-aging nutrients, you will start to see results in as little as two to three weeks.

Q. What if I'm stuck at work or on the road, and can't juice or blend?

A. Purchase an all-organic juice blend powder you can mix on the go. If not available, simply choose foods that are healthy and free from chemicals or toxins. Jamba Juice and Starbucks both carry organic juice blends.

Q. Can I take vitamins (i.e. a multi vitamin)?

A. If you are getting the recommended daily servicing of fruits and vegetables, vitamins are a waste of money and often cause more problems then they solve. Seek alternative options like organic supplements.

Q. What if the food label says natural?

A. Most food companies are deceptive in marketing their

products to consumers in the hope that they will buy. A good practice is to read the label. Unless it says "organic," if it lists ingredients that sound like chemicals, avoid it. Food manufacturers are not required by law to list all the chemicals or ingredients in their products.

Q. Do I really need to be that concerned about products I put on my skin?

A. Yes, yes, and yes. The skin is the largest organ and the most absorbent, so always choose organic, all-natural products when applying creams to your skin or brushing your teeth or dying your hair. The goal is to eliminate a large percentage of toxins from your daily intake. If you don't achieve this, nothing will change, and you will continue to look the same, feel the same, and act the same.

Q. What about eating in restaurants?

A. Restaurants are about flavor, and often use all types of age-robbing chemicals and fats to make their products taste great and addictive. Be mindful of what goes into the food and only choose raw, organic options. If unavailable, enjoy, then get back to your routine of eating and juicing organic 80% of the time.

Q. Must I really take a daily probiotic?

A. Yes. A balanced gut is 60%-70% of your appearance and health. Without it, your food cravings will go thought the roof and your health and appearance will suffer. Healthy gut bacteria are your greatest appearance and health advocates.

Q. Do I really need to consult with my doctor?

A. It's always a good idea to mention or bring my book in to your doctor, especially if you're taking medications. Some foods or herbs may have a negative effect on some drugs. So it's a good idea to give your doctor the list of superfoods mentioned in the book to make sure there aren't any problems.

Q. *Is it a good idea to add plant-based protein powers to my juice or blend?*

A. Yes. Proteins are essential in feeding our cells, brains, and making hormones.

Q. *Can I juice all day long?*

A. For a day or two when detoxing, but remember that skipping meals, even when juicing, can make you feel moody, tired, and hungry, often sabotaging good food choices. Our brains need protein for our neurons to make chemical endorphins that make us feel calm and happy. Blood sugar irregularities due to a lack of protein put the body into flight or fight mode, increasing depression and anxiety.

Q. *How much fruit should I use in juicing or blending?*

A. Many people get carried away with the taste of the juice or smoothie, so they load up on the fruits, which creates a concentrated source of natural sugar that spikes insulin. Not good. The goal is to be balanced. So the rule is 80% veggies and 20% fruits high in sugar like carrots, pineapple, mango, papaya, and banana.

Q. *Do I really need to wash my produce even if it's organic?*

A. Yes. Don't skip this step for either organic or conventional. Either wash or use a potato peeler to take off the first layer, then wash and cut off any ends. For example, apples should always be quartered, carrots peeled, etc.

Q. *Will I really see wrinkles diminish, healthier skin, hair, and nails?*

A. Yes. This is the exciting part. Your body *wants* to heal itself and regenerate cells. When you remove toxins, balance out the good bacteria in your gut and flood your cells with fresh organic building materials to replace old, weak, and diseased ones. Your energy levels will return, and your health and appreciate will noticeably improve, in as little as thirty days post-detox.

Q. How long should I detox before I start the anti-aging juice blends?

A. It depends on how long you've been living a toxic lifestyle. The average person should be detox for a minimum of two to three weeks. This means eliminating processed foods, drinking detox juicing blends daily, taking your probiotic, and following the detox steps laid out in the book. It takes some clients up to a month to replace toxic products they use with natural ones, clean up their habits, and eliminate their toxin overload.

Q. Can I juice or blend and drink it later?

A. Yes, but only if you freeze it in ice cube trays. Plant nutrition is volatile and unstable, and juicing or blending tears cell walls open to release nutrients. That's why juice needs to be consumed as soon as possible. Oxidation can lead to loss of important nutritional components like iron, zinc, and magnesium. So it's best to drink it once you've made it, or freeze it.

Q. Do I really need to get a shower filter?

A. Without question. Most skin and health conditions are caused by toxic soaps, creams and chemicals absorbed in showers. The goal of looking and feeling 10 years younger is to remove as many of these toxins as possible, so the body can get back to producing health vibrant resilient cells as opposed to spinning its wheels just keeping you alive in a toxic body. Doing this little thing you will be amazed on the improvement of your skin and hair. Not to mention all the added health benefits you will gain from toxic elimination.

REFERENCES

1. Anderson GH. "Sugars and health: A review". Source: *Nutrition Research* Volume: 17 Issue: 9 Pages: 1485-1498 DOI: 10.1016/S0271-5317(97)00139-5 Published: SEP 1997

2. Johnson, Rachel, Appel, Lawrence, Brands, Michael. "Dietary Sugars Intake and Cardiovascular Health: A Scientific Statement From the American Heart Association." 2009;120:1011-1020, published online before print, August 24 2009, doi:10.1161/CIRCULATIONAHA.109.192627.

3. Price, W— Nutrition and Physical Degeneration 1997

4. Ruxton C. H. S.; Gardner E. J.; McNulty H. M. "Is Sugar Consumption Detrimental to Health? A Review of the Evidence 1995-2006" Source: *Critical Reviews in Food Science and Nutrition* Volume: 50 Issue: 1 Pages: 1-19 Article Number: PII 918157476 DOI: 10.1080/10408390802248569 Published: 2010

5. USDA. "Profiling Food Consumption in America." United States Department of Agriculture. Sowers, Robert. 2010. http://www.usda.gov/factbook/chapter2.pdf.

6. "Role of Sugars in Human Neutrophilic Phagocytosis." *American Journal of Clinical Nutrition*, 1973, 26pp. 1, 180-4).

---

1. Hilary Parker. A sweet problem: Princeton researchers find that high-fructose corn syrup prompts considerably more weight gain. Princeton University. 2010 March 22.

2. American Chemical Society. Soda Warning-high-fructose corn syrup linked to diabetes, new study suggests. *Science Daily* 23 Aug. 2007.

3. Jennifer K. Nelson R.D.,L.D. What is high-fructose corn syrup? What are the health concerns? Mayo Clinic. 2012 September 27.

4. Duke University Medical Center. <u>High fructose corn syrup linked to liver scarring, research suggests</u>. *Science Daily*. 23 Mar. 2010.

5. Laura G. Sánchez-Lozada, Wei Mu, Carlos Roncal, Yuri Y. Sautin, Manal Abdelmalek, Sirirat Reungjui, MyPhuong Le, Takahiko Nakagawa, Hui Y. Lan, Xuequing Yu, Richard J. Johnson. <u>Comparison of free fructose and glucose to sucrose in the ability to cause fatty liver</u>. *European Journal of Nutrition*. 2010 February. vol. 49 issue 1, pp. 1-9.

6. Dufault R, LeBlanc B, Schnoll R, Cornett C, Schweitzer L, Wallinga D, Hightower J, Patrick L, Lukiw WJ. <u>Mercury from chlor-alkali plants: measured concentrations in food product sugar</u>. *Environ Health*. 2009 Jan 26;8:2. doi: 10.1186/1476-069X-8-2.

U.S. Council of Environmental Quality "Drinking tap water that is chlorinated is hazardous, if not deadly to your health."

Healthy Water for a Longer Life

Dr. Martin Fox

"Chlorine is the greatest crippler and killer of modern times. While it prevented epidemics of one disease, it was creating another. Two decades ago, after the start of chlorinating our drinking water in 1904, the present epidemic of heart trouble, cancer and senility began."

Saginaw Hospital

Dr. J.M. Prince, M.D.

"The cause of atherosclerosis and resulting heart attacks and strokes is none other than ubiquitous chlorine in our drinking water."

Coronaries/Cholesterol/Chlorine
Dr. J.M. Prince, M.D.

"In the vast majority of cases where germ-free water is required whether for public supply or in the swimming pool, the process of disinfection will involve the use of chlorine in one form or another."

Chemistry and Control of Modern Chlorination
Dr. A.T. Palin, Ph.D. (O.B.E.)

"A Professor of Water Chemistry at the University of Pittsburg claims that exposure to vaporized chemicals in the water supplies through showering, bating, and inhalation is 100 times greater than through drinking the water."

"As chlorine is added to kill pathogenic microorganisms, the highly reactive chlorine combines with fatty acids and carbon fragments to form a variety of toxic compounds, which comprise about 30% of the chlorination by-products."

"During the mid-1970s, monitoring efforts began to identify wide-spread toxic contamination of the nation s drinking water supplies, epidemiological studies began to suggest a link between ingestion of toxic chemicals in the water and elevated cancer mortality risks. Since those studies were completed, a variety of additional studies have strengthened the statistical connection between consumption of toxins in water and elevated cancer risks. Moreover, this basic concern has been heightened by other research discoveries."

The Nader Report — Troubled Waters On Tap
Center for Study of Responsive Law

"The National Academy of Scientists states that people die in the United States each year from cancers caused by ingesting the contaminants in water. The major health threat posed by these pollutants is far more likely to be from their inhalation as air pollutants. The reason that emissions are high is that water droplets dispersed by the shower head have a larger surface-to-volume ratio than water streaming into the bath."

Science News, Vol, 130

Janet Raloff

"Evidence points to chlorine-based compounds (organochlorines) as significant contributors to the epidemic of chronic illnesses in humans, including breast cancer in women, and reproductive, developmental, immunological, behavioral and endocrine disorders. In addition, chlorine-based chemicals, like CFCs and other refrigerants, are primarily responsible for the destruction of the Earth's protective ozone layer."

Greenpeace. - Jan. Feb. & Mar., 1993

"A long, hot shower can be dangerous. The toxic chemicals are inhaled in high concentrations."

Bottom Line August 87

Dr. Julian Andeiman, Ph.D.

"Skin adsorption of contaminants has been underestimated and ingestion may not consitiute the sole or even primary route of exposure."

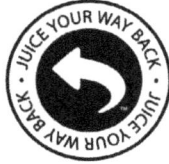

For more information, visit our website:
www.juiceyourwayback.com

For bulk purchases or general questions,
write: info@juiceyourwayback.com

If you enjoyed this book, please share your thoughts by leaving
a review where you purchased the book.
Thank you.

www.ingramcontent.com/pod-product-compliance
Lightning Source LLC
Chambersburg PA
CBHW031510270326
41930CB00006B/344